Praise for *Opening Up by Writing It Down*

"The power of expressing emotions is one of the most important discoveries psychologists have ever made. The authors blend scientific rigor with practical wisdom, in an accessible book chock-full of insights. Write it down!"
  —Shelley E. Taylor, PhD, Distinguished Professor,
  Department of Psychology, University of California, Los Angeles

"An absorbing account of expressive writing and how it works. This book is full of ideas and techniques that will benefit anyone who reads it."
  —Timothy D. Wilson, PhD, author of *Redirect: Changing the Stories We Live By*

"Fascinating. We learn that writing positively affects the immune system and can be a powerful tool in the treatment of trauma, psychological problems, and chronic disease. If you want to jump-start your brain, cleanse the mind, or resolve troublesome experiences, check out this classic book."
  —Susan M. Pollak, MTS, EdD, psychologist, Cambridge, Massachusetts

"*Opening Up by Writing It Down, Third Edition*, is a wonderfully crafted blend of engaging examples and current scientific knowledge. The authors make a compelling case that people can improve their overall health and well-being by writing about troubling feelings and experiences. The book is fun and motivating, and it includes helpful exercises and suggestions to get you started on this path to wellness."
  —Dena Rosenbloom, PhD, author of *Life After Trauma*

OPENING UP BY WRITING IT DOWN

Opening Up by Writing It Down

THIRD EDITION

How Expressive Writing Improves Health
and Eases Emotional Pain

JAMES W. PENNEBAKER, PhD

JOSHUA M. SMYTH, PhD

The Guilford Press
New York   London

3385704

DEC 2 2 2016

Library of Congress Cataloging-in-Publication Data

Names: Pennebaker, James W., author. | Smyth, Joshua M., author.
Title: Opening up by writing it down : how expressive writing improves
    health and eases emotional pain / James W. Pennebaker and Joshua M.
    Smyth.
Other titles: Opening up
Description: Third edition. | New York, NY : The Guilford Press, [2016] |
    Revision of: Opening up / James W. Pennebaker. 1997. | Includes
    bibliographical references and index.
Identifiers: LCCN 2016006014 | ISBN 9781462524921 (paperback : acid-free
    paper)
Subjects: LCSH: Self-disclosure—Health aspects. | Written
    communication—Therapeutic use. | Stress (Psychology)—Prevention. |
    Mind and body. | BISAC: PSYCHOLOGY / Mental Health. | MEDICAL /
    Mental Health. | RELIGION / Counseling. | SOCIAL SCIENCE / Social
    Work.
Classification: LCC RC455.4.I54 P46 2016 | DDC 616.89/165—dc23
LC record available at *http://lccn.loc.gov/2016006014*

Contents

Authors' Note · vii

Introduction · ix

1 "Shh . . . It's a Secret": Beginning to Explore
the Connection between Confession and Health · 1

2 The Invention of the Expressive
Writing Approach · 13

3 What's on Your Mind?: Health Benefits
of Verbal and Written Disclosure · 27

4 Dealing with Chronic Health Problems
Using Expressive Writing · 42

5 Writing to Clear the Mind: Expressive Writing
in Learning and Education · 65

6 "Get These Thoughts Out of My Head!":
Getting Past Obsessions, Insomnia,
and Bouts of Stupidity · 81

7 To Speed Up or Slow Down?: How People Differ
in Coping with Trauma · 96

8 "I'm Here for You . . . or Am I?": The Audience
on the Other End of Our Words · 115

9   How Does Writing Help Us Secure a Healthier   135
    and Happier Future?

10 Pulling It All Together: 158
    Recommendations for Your Use
    of Expressive Writing

    Notes   171

    Bibliography   183

    Author Index   199

    Subject Index   202

    About the Authors   210

Authors' Note

Throughout this book, we refer to individuals we have studied or interviewed. In all cases, we have changed the names and other identifying information about the people involved to protect their anonymity. In addition, we have reconstructed some of the direct spoken quotations from memory or notes of conversations. The gist of each of the stories, however, is true and based on real people.

Introduction

Expressive writing is a technique where people typically write about an upsetting experience for 15 to 20 minutes a day for three or four days. This very simple exercise has been found to improve people's physical and mental health for weeks, months, and even years when compared to individuals who write about emotionally neutral topics (or other comparison groups). The method was first described in a scientific paper in 1986, and since then several hundred expressive writing experiments have been conducted.

Expressive writing is not simply a form of journaling or diary writing. It's not a practice that will help you become a novelist or screenwriter. Rather, it is a brief writing technique that helps people understand and deal with emotional upheavals in their lives. It is a little like a self-help therapy without outlandish claims. Its greatest appeal is that it is a method with strong scientific evidence behind it.

This book was written with two audiences in mind. The first includes people who may be dealing with a difficult personal situation who want to know more about ways to get through a tough time. The second group of readers includes those who are simply curious about expressive writing and how it works. We hope that we motivate current or prospective students, colleagues, and laypeople to think more about the fascinating topics surrounding expressive writing.

The original editions of the book were published in 1990 and 1997. So much has happened since the earlier editions. A more complete story was needed for a broader audience. Expressive writing has been used to treat a variety of physical health problems as well as mental health issues such as anxiety, depression, and posttraumatic stress disorder (or PTSD). We've learned that expressive writing improves college adjustment and results in better grades. It even helps people's relationships and love lives.

But, as you will see, writing doesn't work with everyone. The effects are typically modest but usually beneficial, helping people across cultures and circumstances. In this edition, we offer opportunities to try it yourself in different ways. We still don't have a solid explanation of why it does and doesn't work—although we are getting some better ideas. The writing research community is made up of clinical, social, health, and cognitive psychologists; social workers; physicians; and even the occasional person in business and education.

The expressive writing world is far more complex and dynamic today than it was 30 years ago when Jamie Pennebaker first described the early findings. The current book has a far greater reach because of the collaboration with Joshua Smyth. Whereas Jamie was the inventor of the method, Josh advanced the field through his hard-nosed experiments and concise scientific mind. The two of us have worked closely together to bring a much more modern and, we hope, balanced view to the expressive writing literature.

We similarly hope you find this book both honest and helpful. Although we are convinced that expressive writing can be a valuable tool, we are not "true believers." There isn't any one way to write. What works for some people may not work for you. By seeing the different ways that writing has worked in research studies, we hope you might be encouraged to try writing on your own.

Above all, we encourage you to become your own scientist. If you, a friend, or a client is plagued with unwanted thoughts, memories, or worries, expressive writing may be helpful. If it isn't helpful, try writing in some different ways. If it still doesn't help you, try other avenues—therapy, exercise, meditation, or something else. Experiment, experiment, experiment.

A book such as this is ultimately a joint work of hundreds of people. We are humbled by the colleagues, editors, therapists, students, and practitioners who have influenced our thinking and, more generally, the direction our research has taken us. More immediately, the research on which this book is based was conducted with the help of thousands of participants—some healthy college students and others suffering from disease or other painful life circumstances. To conduct these studies, we have often relied on the help and collaboration of an amazing group of graduate and undergraduate students over the last three decades. Finally, we thank our family and friends for sharing their lives with us while we lost ourselves in our labs. We are deeply grateful and indebted to all of you.

We hope you enjoy reading about the experiments others have tried and that they can inform your studies on yourself.

CHAPTER 1

"Shh . . . It's a Secret"

BEGINNING TO EXPLORE THE CONNECTION
BETWEEN CONFESSION AND HEALTH

Why do people around the world tell their stories? Is there some kind of urge to confess? Is it healthy for us to divulge our deepest thoughts and feelings? Or, conversely, is it unhealthy *not* to share the private sides of our lives with others? Questions such as these have captivated psychologists, anthropologists, journalists, and others for generations. This book tells the story about the nature of secrets, self-disclosure, and health. It started with a number of personal twists and turns in our own lives; yet, as we explored these topics, family, friends, students, and colleagues joined in. Their stories, too, are woven throughout this book.

Major secrets can be stressful.* Like other stressors, keeping secrets from those close to us can affect our health, including our immune function, the action of our heart and vascular systems, and even the biochemical workings of our brain and nervous systems. In short, keeping back thoughts, feelings, and behaviors can place us at risk for both major and minor diseases.

Whereas harboring secrets is potentially harmful, confronting our personal thoughts and feelings can have remarkable short- and long-term health benefits. Confession, whether by writing or talking

---

*This will be the only footnote you will see in the book. Rather than break up the story, we have included references and additional information in the Notes section at the end of the book.

(or many other forms of emotional expression or disclosure, as we will see throughout the book), can neutralize many of the problems of secrets. Talking or writing about upsetting things can influence our basic values, our daily thinking patterns, and our feelings about ourselves. In fact, there appears to be a basic need to reveal ourselves to others. Not disclosing our thoughts and feelings can be risky for our mental and physical health. Divulging them can be healthy.

These are the most basic ideas of the book. But, there is much more to the story. Before detailing the nature of revealing secrets, it's helpful to explain how we got into this business.

Setting the Stage: Clues to the Links among Secrets, Disclosure, and Health

You will notice that there are two authors of this book: Jamie Pennebaker and Josh Smyth. We have each taken our own journey as it relates to this work. Our stories are quite a bit different, but they both point to the ways almost-random experiences can set up lifelong career paths. Both of us were originally trained as social psychologists—people who study, among other things, attitudes, behaviors, and everyday social relationships. A strong and persistent interest for both of us is how people choose to share their personal experiences with others.

THE JOY OF TALKING

Early in his career, Jamie became fascinated by three seemingly unrelated phenomena: the joy of talking, the nature of lie detection, and the role of self-understanding in influencing the mind–body link (particularly as it related to health and well-being). Piecing together these observations laid the groundwork of an intriguing model that would help map out the nature and consequences of holding secrets and confronting emotional experiences. After graduate school, Jamie found himself teaching a class of 300 freshmen about basic psychology. One day, as part of a class demonstration, he split the students into small groups of people who didn't know one another. Once in their assigned groups, the students were told just to talk for 15 minutes about anything they wanted. As you would expect, they talked about their hometowns, why they had come to college, what dormitory they lived in, friends they had in common, the weather, and related topics—the usual cocktail party fare.

At the end of 15 minutes, everyone returned to their regular seats and estimated how much of the time every person in the group had talked, how much they liked the group, and how much they had learned from the group. Two rather surprising findings emerged:

- *The more people talked, the more they liked the group.*
- *The more they themselves talked, the more they claimed to have learned from the group.*

In other words, as a group member, the more you dominate the conversation, the more you claim that you have learned about the others. In general, it seems we would rather talk than listen. Most of us find that communicating our thoughts is a supremely enjoyable learning experience.

THE POLYGRAPH CONFESSION EFFECT

As you'll see later in the book, both of us have long been fascinated by the links between people's emotions and their physiological activity. An important formative experience occurred when one of us was introduced to the world of lie detection—in particular, the use of biological clues to determine when people were not being truthful.

There is something frighteningly magical about the idea of lie detection. Machines that can accurately read others' private thoughts have been the basis of dreams by police officers, poker players, and parents. A crude approximation of this magical lie detector is the polygraph—an instrument that continuously measures several physiological indicators such as heart rate, blood pressure, breathing rate, and perspiration on the hand.

In law enforcement, polygraph exams and related lie detection methods assume that when suspects try to deceive their interrogators, their biological stress levels will increase relative to when they tell the truth. In other words, telling a lie should be stressful, and we should be able to reliably detect this response. Although polygraph techniques do better than chance at catching truly guilty suspects, they are far from perfect.

The real value of the polygraph is in bringing about confessions. A particularly skilled polygrapher uses a suspect's biological responses to various questions as an indicator of what topics provoke the most anxiety. Once the "hot" questions are isolated, the polygrapher may note, "Gee, I really believe what you have told me, but my machine shows a huge reaction when you answered that question. Why do you think this is happening?" In more cases than not, deceptive suspects try to rationalize their physiological responses. In so doing, they often contradict their earlier stories. The more they are confronted with these contradictions, the more likely they are to ultimately break down and confess to the crime.

In the early 1980s, Jamie was invited to give a series of talks on emotion and health to some of the top-level polygraphers of the FBI, CIA, and other secret agencies. He spent several late evenings talking with the polygraphers about their jobs. As a group, these people were unusually bright and insightful. Most impressive was a remarkably similar experience that many of the polygraphers reported in interrogating some of their suspects—something we call the *polygraph confession effect*.

A San Francisco–based polygrapher gave an unforgettable account of the polygraph confession effect. He was called in to give a polygraph exam to a 45-year-old bank vice president who was a suspect in an embezzlement investigation. When initially run through the polygraph exam, the bank vice president's heart rate, blood pressure, and other physiological levels were quite high. This is normal for both innocent and guilty people because such an exam is almost always threatening. Nevertheless, the polygrapher suspected that the bank vice president was lying or holding back information because his physiological levels went even higher when the vice president was asked about some of the details of the embezzlement. With repeated questions and prodding, the vice president finally broke down and confessed to embezzling $74,000 over a six-month period.

In line with standard procedures, after the bank vice president had signed a written confession, he was polygraphed again to be certain that his confession was itself not deceptive. When tested the second time, his overall physiological levels were extremely low. His hands were no longer sweaty. His heart rate and blood pressure were extraordinarily low. His breathing was slow and relaxed.

You can appreciate the irony of this situation. This man had come into the polygrapher's office a free man, safe in the knowledge that polygraph evidence was not allowed in court. Nevertheless, he confessed. Now, his professional, financial, and personal life was on the brink of ruin. He was virtually assured of a prison term. Despite these realities, he was relaxed and at ease with himself. Later, when a policeman came to handcuff and escort him to jail, he warmly shook the polygrapher's hand and thanked him for all he had done. Several months later, the polygrapher received a warm Christmas card written by the former bank vice president with the federal penitentiary as the return address.

Even when the costs are high, the confession of painful secrets can reduce anxiety and physiological stress. Whereas being the center of the conversation in a group may be fun, revealing pent-up thoughts and feelings can be liberating—even if they end up sending you to prison.

PSYCHOSOMATICS, SELF-KNOWLEDGE, AND HEALING

Here's a little tip about researchers in psychology: Many of them study topics that are most troublesome or relevant for them personally. It is possible that Jamie was interested in emotion and health issues because of family issues earlier in his life. He was probably drawn to the area of psychosomatics by virtue of having had asthma as a child. He grew up in West Texas, a very dry and flat part of the world. During his adolescence, asthma attacks became a routine feature of the windy part of winter (as opposed to the windy parts of spring, summer, and fall). At the time, he reasoned that pollen and dust that had blown in from New Mexico and Nevada were to blame.

In college, he never had any wheezing bouts except when he went home for the Christmas holidays. The pollen and dust again. During his last year in college, however, his parents came to visit him in Florida in late November. The day they arrived, he developed asthma. All of a sudden, the profound realization hit him that there was more to asthma than pollen. We don't want to be judgmental here, but one could reasonably argue that long-standing conflicts with his parents were linked to his upper respiratory system. Interestingly, once he saw the parent–asthma connection, he never wheezed again. It was far too embarrassing.

For Josh it was a bit different. He was an independent and autonomous child. He had a highly active fantasy life, largely fueled by a great love of reading. In particular, he loved more fantastical books—

fairy tales, superheroes, mythology, that kind of stuff. This fascina-
tion persisted for years and curiously matched up with some college
studies years later. During college, Josh took a course that covered,
among other things, mind–body processes. That is, how the mind
could exert influence over the body—think mind over matter, resist-
ing pain, controlling heart rate and other automatic biological functions, and so forth. This was tantamount to the paranormal themes
that had always been so captivating for him. It almost sounds like
a superpower, doesn't it? But it raised thorny issues: How could the
mind influence our physical bodies? How could some cells, some particularly important bits in our brains presumably, control all the other
squishy bits in our bodies? From this point on, Josh was hooked—he
had to figure out how our minds could influence our bodies.

You can already see the beginnings of what will be part of the
larger story—personal experiences, insights, sometimes even formal
research, can each lead to observations on how things work. These
observations lead to careful exploration using scientific methods, and
this cycle continues over time as understanding grows. In many ways,
this is the essence of science in general, and certainly has been a central theme in exploring the links between psychological experiences
and our health and well-being.

Psychological Links to Illness and Health

Asthma, wheezing, congestion, and other respiratory changes have
long been known to be related to psychological conflict. In fact, in the
mid-20th century Harold G. Wolff and Stewart Wolf, two pioneers in
the emerging field known as psychosomatic medicine, explored the
links between people's psychological conflicts and health problems
in books with intriguing titles such as *The Nose* (together and sepa-
rately, they also published books entitled *Headache, The Colon,* and, of
course, *The Stomach*). In landmark studies spanning three decades,
Wolff, Wolf, and their collaborators developed the stress interview,
whereby volunteers would be asked a series of psychologically threatening questions while, at the same time, relevant bodily changes were
monitored.

The stress interview serves as a medical version of a lie detector
exam. For most people, there are a limited number of psychological

issues that account for most psychosomatic problems. Current stress interviews, for example, routinely touch on issues of loss, rejection, sexuality, parental problems, uncontrollable trauma, and failure. Depending on the person's health problem, the interviewer might measure muscle tension in the neck (for tension headache sufferers), blood pressure and heart rate (for people with hypertension), breathing rate or oxygen consumption (for those with respiratory problems or panic attacks), or one of a few dozen other biological indices.

As Wolff, Wolf, and a generation of psychosomatic researchers asserted, psychological conflicts are sometimes linked to specific changes in our bodies. One person's blood pressure may increase when he is forced to discuss the death of his parents, whereas another might respond to the same topic with the beginnings of a migraine headache. A third person may not show any biological changes in response to the death topic but may react selectively to issues surrounding sexuality.

That many, perhaps most, illnesses have a psychosomatic component is not surprising. More peculiar is that we rarely see the relationship between psychological events and illness in ourselves. When we do, however, the course of the illness often changes for the better.

Why are we blind to many of the psychological precursors to illness? One problem lies in our abilities to perceive cause–effect relationships. When we see something happen, we naturally look for something that preceded the event by no more than a few seconds or, at most, hours. If our car doesn't start because of a dead battery, we might blame the battery's demise on last night's cold weather or our failure to turn off the headlights. It makes no sense to think back to the way we drove the car two weeks ago. Our body is a different story. If we come down with a cold, it probably has nothing to do with last night's weather or what we had for breakfast. It could be that our immune system was compromised by the breakup of a significant relationship a week or two earlier.

Another reason for our inability to see the links between our own psychological issues and illness concerns denial. Virtually all of us have actively avoided thinking about unpleasant experiences. Some issues are so painful that we deceive ourselves into thinking that they don't exist. Sigmund Freud persuasively argued that we employ an arsenal of defense mechanisms, such as denial, compulsive behaviors, and even dwelling on physical symptoms to screen out anxiety and psychological pain. Wheezing when around parents or headaches in sexual situations can safely be attributed to purely physical causes (e.g., pollen or caffeine). Admitting to personal struggles concerning one's autonomy or feelings of sexual anxiety is a far less pleasant strategy when less threatening alternative explanations are available.

Fortunately, once we become aware of the psychological causes of a recurring health problem such as headaches, back pain, or asthma, the problems often subside to some degree. There are several reasons for this. Once we see the psychological basis for a particular health problem, we can use the health problem as a signal of distress. By focusing our energy on reducing the cause of the distress, we more quickly resolve the underlying psychological issues that we may not have known were issues in the first place. Another reason that seeing the cause–effect relationship is beneficial is that it makes the health problems more predictable and, hence, controllable. Perceptions of control and predictability over our worlds are essential to good psychological health.

A recurring debate among researchers interested in psychosomatics and emotion concerns whether specific emotions or situations can bring about specific biological changes. Our bias is that many emotions do, in fact, have necessary and potentially unique biological substrates. However, particularly powerful situations can "fool" people into thinking that they are feeling an emotion that is not biologically present.

A good example of this often invisible link between a psychological event and biological activity occurred with Warren, an extremely bright student who had been the valedictorian of his high school class. After performing quite well his first year and a half of college, he suddenly developed test anxiety. Midway through his second year of college, he began to fail every test he took. He was soon placed on academic probation and later forced to withdraw from school. Over the next year, Warren saw a therapist who specialized in behavioral treatments. Several weeks of relaxation training and behavior modification failed to produce significant improvements.

Two years after his problems started, Warren explained his predicament. He agreed to be interviewed about his life while his heart rate was continuously measured. During the first hour-long interview, it became clear that Warren's body was telling a different story than Warren's words.

Topic	Heart rate	Warren's comments
Girlfriend	77	Fairly new relationship. Some conflict about sex, but we're close.
College courses	71	Most have been interesting . . . tests have been another matter.
Failing exams	76	It's been hard on my ego. I can't explain it.
Parents	84	We were a close family until the divorce.
Parents' divorce	103	It was no big deal, really. They are a lot happier now.
The future	79	It scares me. I can't bear the thought of failing again.

Look at how Warren's heart rate jumped dramatically whenever the topic of his parents' divorce was discussed. No other issues influenced his heart rate to a comparable degree. Despite the fact that Warren claimed to be unaffected by his parents' divorce, his striking physiological responses to this topic suggest that it was a significant event. Indeed, he first learned that they had separated about a week before his developing test anxiety. As an only child, he had rarely spoken about it with anyone. In fact, he had kept the divorce secret from his previous girlfriend because he felt it was a private matter. In the two intervening years, he never saw the relationship between the divorce and his poor performance during exams. When confronted with his heart rate data, Warren was flabbergasted. Over the next few days, he discussed his feelings of anger and despair over the divorce with Jamie and, later, with his parents and his current girlfriend. Although he still harbored some of these feelings, his test anxiety disappeared.

We are often blind to the psychological causes and correlates of our health problems. Many illnesses and recurring health problems have a psychosomatic component. Awareness of or insight into the psychological bases of our illnesses can benefit us. If we are aware of the conflicts influencing our bodies, we can act to overcome those conflicts. We are very good at fooling ourselves. People often fail to see a cause–effect relation between a psychological event and an illness because they do not *want* to see it. You can appreciate the paradox. To

not see something that is threatening requires some degree of awareness that the threatening event or relation exists.

Fitting the Puzzle Together

These were the beginning pieces of the puzzle. When we talk a great
deal in a group, we claim that we enjoy it and learn from it. After
confessing a crime, our minds and bodies appear to be relaxed. Once
we understand the link between a psychological event and a recurring
health problem, our health improves.

Each of these phenomena deals with the psychological state of
holding back versus letting go. You can begin to see the organizing
framework. Although it is still evolving, it can be summarized as follows:

• *Keeping secrets is physical work.* When we try to keep a secret,
we must actively hold back or inhibit our thoughts, feelings, or behaviors. Keeping secrets from others means that we must consciously
restrain, hold back, or in some way exert effort to *not* think, feel, or
behave.

• *Secrets can produce short-term biological changes and influence long-term health.* In the short run, restraining thoughts or feelings can immediately affect our body, for example, by increasing
perspiration or causing faster heart rates, as seen during lie detector
tests. Over time, the work of keeping secrets serves as a cumulative
stressor on the body, increasing the likelihood of illness and other
stress-related physical and mental problems. Actively holding back
from talking about important topics is one of many general stressors
that affect the mind and body. The harder we must work at hiding our
thoughts or feelings, the greater the stress on our bodies.

• *Secrets hurt our thinking abilities.* Actively holding back can
disrupt the ways we think. If we don't talk about a powerfully emotional experience with others, it's almost impossible to organize it in
our minds in a broad and integrative way. When keeping a big secret,
we don't translate the event into language. This can prevent us from
understanding the event. Major life experiences that are withheld
from others are likely to surface in the forms of anxiety, ruminations,
disturbing dreams, and other thought disturbances.

The human mind naturally tries to understand the world around it. One reason we often obsess about a disturbing experience is that we are trying to understand it. An efficient way to understanding something is to talk about it—to translate it into words. If we don't talk about it, we continue to think about it. And if we keep ruminating about it, we have fewer mental resources to think about other things. This helps explain why people under stress often have memory problems and are less attentive to changes in themselves and others.

• *Disclosure reduces the effects of secrets.* The act of disclosing a trauma reduces the physiological work of secrets. During disclosure, the biological stress of holding back is immediately reduced. Over time, if we continue to confront and thereby resolve our emotional upheavals, there will be a lowering of our overall stress level.

• *Disclosure forces a rethinking of events.* Disclosing or confronting a trauma helps us understand and ultimately assimilate the event. By talking or writing about a secret experience, we are translating the event into language. Once it is language based, we can better understand the experience and ultimately put it behind us.

Casting a 21st-Century Spin on Some Old Ideas

Early theories by Aristotle, and more recent elaborations by Josef Breuer and Sigmund Freud, suggested that circumstances that prevent people from disclosing emotional experiences will lead to hysterical symptoms. Freud suggested that there may be a human need for some kind of catharsis. He and Breuer came up with the idea of having people talk about their thoughts and emotions as a way of curing mental distress. Their "talking cure" was later incorporated into several modern approaches to psychotherapy.

Despite the work by Freud and several contemporary psychologists, many of our colleagues have viewed the secret/confession/catharsis approach as a bit extreme and even radical. Others have found it a novel and stimulating topic. Given the polarized reception of the early work, both of us knew there was something interesting and potentially important to be explored.

After conducting one of the early experiments on secrets, health, and disclosure, Jamie was thrilled by the patterns of effects he was finding. Soon after an exciting meeting with his students, Jamie waltzed in the front door of his home just as his phone rang. His brother, who is a graphic designer, called to ask what was new. Jamie excitedly told him about this new approach to studying secrets, inhibition, and disclosure and its possible links to health, psychotherapy, religion, and, well, just about everything. Not swayed by his grandiosity, his brother asked about the specifics of the emerging framework. When Jamie was finished, the phone was silent. "That's it?" his brother finally said. "What's the big deal? Everyone knows *that*."

He was, of course, right on a certain level. We do know that talking about our problems can be good for us. But we also quite often get the sense that we should put on a happy face and look at everything in a positive light. We also know that whining and complaining about our problems will nearly always get us nowhere, or even make things worse. In other words, in these days of self-help popular psychology, we often encounter pithy but contradictory bits of wisdom about how to live your life.

Delve into the self-help literature and you will find that there are gurus and experts who can explain everything to make your life better. And yet their solutions often contradict one another wildly. As our scientific journey into the secret/confrontation world began, we quickly learned that some commonsense ideas were more true than others—indeed, some appeared to be completely false or mistaken. The remainder of this book will share with you some of the insights of this journey and describe some of the interesting discoveries and pitfalls we have encountered on the way.

CHAPTER 2

The Invention of the Expressive Writing Approach

*I*t would be so compelling to tell the story of how the first studies on expressive writing grew out of our traumatic experiences in our childhoods and how we independently discovered the healing power of writing on our own. It would be gripping, initially heartbreaking, and ultimately redemptive. But also false. The expressive writing method was actually the result of a series of serendipitous research findings. Okay, maybe not gripping, but still an interesting story.

The Case of Traumatic Sexual Experiences

Early in his career, Jamie and his students were putting together a questionnaire on health issues. The idea was to break out of the traditional way of thinking and simply ask a large group of students a broad range of questions about their lives. In putting together the questions, the group decided to ask about people's childhoods, their favorite foods, maybe even color preferences. One member of Jamie's research team suggested that they include an item on traumatic sexual experiences in childhood. There was no specific reason for including the question—but it was a question no one appeared to have asked before, and it made intuitive sense that such experiences might be important. So, toward the end of the 12-page questionnaire, they added a question that very few researchers ever ask:

"Prior to the age of 17, did you have a traumatic sexual experience (e.g., rape, being molested)? Yes _____   No _____"

Of the 800 college women who later completed the survey, about 10 percent answered in the affirmative. Overall, the women who reported traumatic sexual experiences in childhood did not differ from others in terms of age, social class, race, or even number of close friends. Most striking, however, was that those who reported a sexual trauma evidenced more health problems than any other group we had ever seen.

Soon afterward, a writer for the magazine *Psychology Today*—one of the most popular magazines of the early 1980s—was able to get 24,000 adults to complete a health survey that included the traumatic sexual experience question. Overall, 22 percent of the women and 10 percent of the men reported having a childhood traumatic sexual experience. These rates roughly corresponded with those found in numerous national polls on the topic.

Even though the reported sexual trauma had occurred almost 20 years earlier, it was associated with large increases in ulcers, the flu, heart problems, cancer diagnoses, and virtually every other category of health problem. In fact, those who reported a traumatic sexual experience as a child had been hospitalized *nearly twice as often* as those who did not report such traumas.

On the *Psychology Today* questionnaire, respondents were asked to include their name and telephone number for possible future telephone interviews. Fifteen people who claimed to have experienced a sexual trauma were called by Carin Rubenstein, the author of the magazine piece. In her article, she writes:

> One woman was raped at 16; another was a victim of incest at 8; yet another had been fondled at the age of 5 by a man selling ponies. A 51-year-old woman from Los Angeles told me that she had been raped, at 5, by her neighbor, who was a friend of the family . . . "I never told anyone about it. You're the first," she said. Later on, not making the connection, she remarked, "I've always had health problems with organs in that area . . . since I was 5." (p. 34)

Every person with whom Rubenstein talked reported an experience that all of us would agree was traumatic. In addition, the majority had not discussed this traumatic event with anyone when it had occurred. If they eventually did discuss their trauma, it was not until many months or years later.

What makes sexual traumas so devastating?

It is clear that childhood sexual traumas influence long-term health. However, changes in health following the traumas may not reflect sexuality per se. Rather, traumas may be insidious because people often cannot talk about them. They must actively inhibit their wanting to discuss these intensely important personal experiences with others.

Later surveys from thousands of people—both students and nonstudents—supported this. Having nearly any kind of traumatic experience is bad for your health. However, if you keep the trauma secret, it increases the odds that you will have health problems. Not surprising, of all the traumas we have studied (death of a family member, victim of violence, moving, failure, personal losses, etc.), people are typically least likely to talk about a sexual trauma.

Expressive Writing and Illness Prevention

If secrets are so bad for us, would talking to others bring about benefits to our health? In the mid-1980s, psychotherapists began providing the first solid research evidence that therapy was good for both mental and physical health. In fact, there had been a couple of largely overlooked insurance studies showing that when insurance companies started coverage for psychotherapy, the extent of and costs associated with physical health care dropped.

What if we set up an experiment where we had people come into the lab and talk to someone about their secret traumatic experiences? You can immediately see the problems with such a study. Where would we find people who would be willing to come in and talk to some stranger about their darkest secrets? Even if we found them, would they really be willing to come to a lab for this? And who should they talk to? How should the people listening to the traumas react? This was too complicated.

And it was about this time that Jamie recalled an experience of his own that had happened eight years earlier. About three years after their wedding, he and his wife were dealing with some formidable issues in their marriage. For the first time in his life, he was despondent, even depressed. Even though he was a graduate student in psychology, he never considered going to a therapist. Instead, after a couple of weeks, he started writing. He wrote about their relationship, his career, his childhood, basically everything that was important to him. In almost no time, the clouds parted. He realized how central his wife was to his very existence.

Recalling this experience, Jamie realized that he could have people write about upheavals in their lives rather than talk to others. Plus, writing would be much simpler to do in an experimental setting.

And so the expressive writing paradigm was born.

The Origin of Expressive Writing

Together with a new graduate student, Sandra Beall, Jamie outlined the following study: The plan was to recruit a group of college students to write about either traumatic experiences or superficial topics. With the students' permission, the student health center would release the number of illness visits each student made in the months before versus after the experiment.

On how many occasions should people write? How long should each writing session last? There was no blueprint for this. Because only a certain number of rooms were available between 5:00 and 10:00 P.M. for four consecutive days, the arithmetic was easy. Jamie and Sandy could run the required number of students if each person wrote for 15 minutes on each of four days. (There is an irony here. People often ask why expressive writing is typically designed to be done for 15 minutes on four days. The answer is that the first study arbitrarily used this approach and it worked, and this approach has been routinely copied since that time.)

On the day of the experiment, students came into a small office. After the study was described and students gave their consent, those assigned to write about their thoughts and feelings about a trauma were told the following:

> "Once you are escorted into the writing cubicle and the door is closed, I want you to write continuously about the most upsetting or traumatic experience of your entire life. Don't worry about grammar, spelling, or sentence structure. In your writing, I want you to discuss your deepest thoughts and feelings about the experience. You can write about anything you want. But whatever you choose, it should be something that

has affected you very deeply. Ideally, it should be something you have not talked about with others in detail. It is critical, however, that you let yourself go and touch those deepest emotions and thoughts that you have. In other words, write about what happened and how you felt about it, and how you feel about it now. Finally, you can write on different traumas during each session or the same one over the entire study. Your choice of trauma for each session is entirely up to you."

Those in the comparison or control group were asked to write about superficial or irrelevant topics during each session. For example, on different days they were asked to describe in detail such things as their dorm room or the shoes they were wearing. The two groups were in the same location, interacting with the same experimenters, and engaging in the activity of writing for the same amount of time; what differed was the content of writing—one group wrote about their deepest thoughts and feelings, and the comparison group wrote about emotionally neutral (and likely quite uninteresting) topics. Thus, the purpose of the control group was to evaluate what effect writing in an experiment per se had on health changes, independent of what was believed to be the important contribution of the content of the writing. Any differences between the two groups should, therefore, be due to the *content* of the writing, not any aspects of their participation in the study.

For the students, the immediate impact of the study was far more powerful than we had ever imagined. Several of the students cried while writing about traumas. Many reported dreaming or continually thinking about their writing topics over the four days of the study. Most telling, however, were the actual writing samples. Essay after essay revealed people's deepest feelings and most intimate sides. Many of the stories depicted profound human tragedies.

One student recounted how his father took him into the backyard on a hot summer night and coolly announced his plans to divorce and move to another town. Although the student was only nine years old at the time, he vividly remembers his father's voice: "Son, the problem with me and your mother was having kids in the first place. Things haven't been the same since you and your sister's birth."

On all four days of the experiment, one woman detailed how, at age 10, her mother asked her to pick up her toys because her grandmother was visiting that evening. She didn't pick up her toys. That night, her grandmother arrived, slipped on one of the toys, and broke her hip. The grandmother died a week later during hip surgery. Now, eight years later, the woman still blamed herself every day.

Another woman described being seduced by her grandfather when she was 13. She depicted the terrible conflict she experienced. On one hand she admitted the physical pleasure of his touching her and the love she felt for her grandfather. On the other, she suffered with the knowledge that this was wrong, that he was betraying her trust.

Other essays disclosed the torture of a woman not able to tell her parents about her being a lesbian, a young man's feelings of loss about the death of his dog, or the anger about parents' divorces. Family abuse, alcoholism, suicide attempts, and public humiliation were also frequent topics.

That a group of college students had experienced so many horrors and, at the same time, had so readily revealed them was remarkable. The grim irony is that, by and large, these were 18-year-old kids attending an upper-middle-class college with above-average high school grades and good College Board scores. These were the people who were portrayed as growing up in the bubble of financial security and suburban tranquility. What must it portend for those brought up in more hostile environments?

The results of the study were fascinating, but also a bit unexpected. Compared to people in the control group, we found that people who wrote about traumatic experience evidenced:

• *Immediate increases in feelings of sadness and anxiety after writing.* Students likened it to the feelings that they had after watching a sad movie. Writing about emotional topics does not produce some kind of immediate release or euphoria.

• *Long-term drops in visits to the student health center for illness.* Those who wrote about emotional upheavals had half the number of illness-related visits to the health center in the six months after the study than people in the control condition.

• *Greater sense of value and meaning as a result of writing.* Not only did people express this in questionnaires afterward, but students would sometimes stop Jamie on campus and thank him for letting them be in the experiment.

The overall pattern of results was exciting. But for every question that the experiment had answered, a dozen more questions appeared.

Perhaps the most basic issue concerned the trustworthiness of these findings. Were the effects real? Does writing about traumas really affect physical health? Perhaps the experiment had just affected people's decisions to visit the student health center. Or even worse, maybe the findings were simply due to chance. Every now and then, for example, you can toss a coin ten times and come up with heads every time.

Additional studies needed to be conducted.

Freewriting

As a useful practice exercise, and one that can enhance creativity and foster your capacity for expression, find a quiet time and place to practice writing. For this exercise, write whatever comes into your mind for 10 to 20 minutes. Try to write the entire time without stopping. Don't worry about style or grammar; the important thing is to keep writing continuously for the entire session. Just let yourself write, a sort of limbering-up exercise. We will return to more structured expressive writing later in the book.

Exploring the Immune System: Writing about Traumas Is Better Than We Thought

Soon after the first expressive writing study was submitted, Jamie teamed up with Janice Kiecolt-Glaser, a clinical psychologist, and her husband, Ronald Glaser, an immunologist, both with the Ohio State University College of Medicine. In the mid-1980s, they were leaders of a new field called psychoneuroimmunology—the mind–body exploration of how mental states and strong emotions might influence the immune system. Together they were blazing a trail by showing that overwhelming experiences such as divorce, major exams in college, and even strong feelings of loneliness adversely affected immune function. They had recently published an article showing that relaxation therapy among the elderly could improve the action of the immune system.

The work by Jan and Ron was groundbreaking because it relied on techniques that directly measured the action of T-lymphocytes, natural killer cells, and other immune markers in the blood. It made

good sense for Jan, Ron, and Jamie to work together—so they set out
to see if expressive writing could directly influence these direct measures of how the immune system was functioning.

The experiment that they designed together was similar to the
first confession study. Fifty students wrote for 20 minutes a day for
four consecutive days about one of two topics. Half wrote about their
deepest thoughts and feelings concerning a trauma. The remaining
25 students were expected to write about superficial topics. The major
difference was that all the students consented to have their blood
drawn the day before writing, after the last writing session, and again
six weeks later.

As before, the experimental volunteers poured out their hearts in
their writing. The tragedies they disclosed were comparable to those in
the first experiment. Instances of rape, child abuse, suicide attempts,
death, and intense family conflict were common. Again, those who
wrote about traumas initially reported feeling sadder and more upset
each day of writing, relative to those who wrote about superficial topics.

Collecting the blood and measuring immune function was a
novel experience that added to the frenzy. As soon as the blood was
drawn, it was driven to the airport to make the last flight to Jan and
Ron's lab in Columbus, Ohio. Once the blood samples arrived, the people in the immunology lab worked around the clock in an assembly-
line manner. The procedure involved separating the blood cells and
placing a predetermined number of white cells in small petri dishes.
Each dish contained differing amounts of various foreign substances,
called mitogens. The dishes were then incubated for two days to allow
the white blood cells time to divide and proliferate in the presence of
the mitogens.

In the body, there are a number of different kinds of white cells,
or lymphocytes, that serve a regulatory function in the immune system. The cells help govern and coordinate aspects of our immune
responses. T-lymphocytes, for example, can stimulate other lymphocytes to make antibodies. Antibodies, along with parts of the body's
defense system, can identify and kill bacteria and viruses foreign to
the body. These aspects of the immune system help keep us healthy.
The immune measures that were used simulated this bodily process
in the dishes. Just as viruses and bacteria can stimulate the growth
of T-lymphocytes in the body, the mitogens did the same in the labo-

ratory dishes. If the lymphocytes divide at a fast rate in response to the mitogens, we can infer that at least part of the immune system is working quickly and efficiently.

What were the findings? People who wrote about their deepest thoughts and feelings surrounding traumatic experiences evidenced enhanced immune function compared with those who wrote about superficial topics. Although this effect was most pronounced after the last day of writing, it tended to persist six weeks after the study. In addition, it was again observed that health center visits for illness dropped for the people who wrote about traumas compared to those who wrote on the trivial topics.

There were now two experiments that showed similar patterns. Taken together, the studies indicated that writing about traumatic experiences could be beneficial. The effects were not due to simple catharsis or the venting of pent-up emotions. In fact, the people who just blew off steam by venting their feelings without any thoughtful analysis tended to fare worse. Further, both experiments indicated that writing about feelings associated with traumatic experiences was painful in the short term. Virtually no one felt excited, on top of the world, or cheerful immediately after writing about the worst experiences of their lives.

In the surveys sent out several months after the experiments, people were asked to describe what long-term effects, if any, the writing experiment had on them. In sharp contrast to the reports immediately after writing, nearly everyone who wrote about traumas now described the study in positive terms. More important, approximately 80 percent explained the value of the study in terms of insight. Rather than explaining that it felt good to get negative emotions off their chests, the respondents noted how they understood themselves better. Some examples:

It helped me think about what I felt during those times. I never realized how it affected me before.

I had to think and resolve past experiences. . . . One result of the experiment is peace of mind, and a method to relieve emotional experiences. To have to write emotions and feelings helped me understand how I felt and why.

Although I have not talked with anyone about what I wrote, I was finally able to deal with it, work through the pain instead of trying to block it out. Now it doesn't hurt to think about it.

The observations of these people and most others who participated in these early studies are almost breathtaking. They tell us that our own thought and emotional processes can help us heal.

Beyond Health:
Writing and Occupational Survival

The early studies were just the beginning of a research odyssey that has taken the expressive writing literature in several directions. Soon after the results of the immune study were published, Stefanie Spera called. Stefanie was a psychologist with an outplacement company in Dallas. An outplacement company typically works with large corporations in the midst of "downsizing"—a polite way of saying the company was laying off a significant number of employees. The outplacement company offers a variety of services to those who have been laid off, including providing office space, secretarial support, and job-hunting skills.

Stefanie called because a large computer company had laid off about 100 senior engineers four months earlier and not one of them had found a new job. She was curious to know if expressive writing could help speed up these engineers getting new jobs.

Over the next few weeks, a sense of how the layoff had occurred started to emerge. The corporation had never had to lay people off in its history. On a Wednesday morning in January, about 100 people, averaging 52 years of age, were individually called into their supervisor's office and informed that they were being terminated with no possibility of being rehired. The employees, most of whom had been with the company since graduating from college almost 30 years earlier, were then escorted to their workspace by a security guard who watched them clean out their desks. They were then taken to the front door, relieved of their keys and security badges, and bid farewell. No forewarning, no retirement watches.

Six months later, an expressive writing study was under way with almost 50 people. Even though they were a rather embittered and hostile group, they were desperate to try anything that might increase their odds of finding another job.

The basic study was quite simple. Half were asked to write about their deepest thoughts and feelings about getting laid off for 30 minutes a day for five consecutive days. The other half wrote for the same period about how they used their time—a strategy based on "time management" (time management was all the rage at that time in the corporate world, despite little if any actual support for such a technique being helpful). A third group of 22 former employees did not write at all and served as another comparison group.

As with our other studies, those who were asked to write about their thoughts and feelings were extremely open and honest in their writing. Their essays described the humiliation and outrage of losing their jobs as well as more intimate themes—marital problems, illness and death, money concerns, and fears about the future.

The potency of the study was surprising. Within three months, 27 percent of the experimental participants landed jobs compared with less than 5 percent of those in the time management and no-writing comparison groups. By seven months after writing, 53 percent of those who wrote about their thoughts and feelings had jobs compared with only 18 percent of the people in the other conditions. Particularly striking about the study was that the participants in all three conditions had all gone on exactly the same number of job interviews. The only difference was that those who had written about their feelings were offered jobs.

Why did writing about getting laid off help these people find jobs more quickly? The key probably has something to do with the nature of anger. Those who had explored their thoughts and feelings were more likely to have come to terms with their extreme hostility toward their previous employer. Recall that these former employees felt betrayed by their company. Even during the initial interviews, it was difficult to stop them from venting their anger. In all likelihood when most of them went on interviews for new jobs, many would let down their guard and talk about how they were treated unfairly and lash out at their former employer—perhaps quite inappropriately so. Those who had written about their thoughts and feelings, on the other hand, were perhaps more likely to have come to terms with getting laid off and, in the interview, came across as less hostile, more promising job candidates.

Does Writing Work?:
The First Round of Meta-Analyses

The first expressive writing study was published in 1986, and the layoff study came out in 1993. Other labs were now starting to conduct and publish writing studies. Most of the studies worked, but some didn't.

At Stony Brook University, a lab headed by Arthur Stone was beginning to run some interesting writing studies. Arthur was a scientist known for having a critical mind and was keenly capable of finding the flaws and limitations of psychology projects. Unfortunately (or, as it turned out, fortunately), his skeptical eye soon was locked on the expressive writing research. Several of his students were interested in expressive writing work, and one of these was Josh.

At this point, over a dozen studies had been conducted and published in the scientific literature. Josh reasoned that this would be an opportunity to apply a statistical method known as meta-analysis to the expressive writing studies. Put simply, a meta-analysis allows us to examine multiple studies in a cumulative fashion, attempting to find out what the overall message (or finding) is from all the studies collectively. By doing this, we can begin to get a more precise estimate of an effect—in this case, to determine if there was strong evidence that expressive writing was helpful.

In other words, this method could tell us whether or not expressive writing was leading to health improvements relative to writing about emotionally neutral topics. Such an approach can address other important questions as well. Are there particular outcomes that appear to show greater or lesser benefit from writing? For example, does writing work better for physical health outcomes or for depression?

In many ways, Josh was well suited to this task. He had adopted his adviser's skepticism but, at the same time, was not wedded to any particular outcome. Josh had another interest—ways to measure hard, objective outcomes. By way of background, social science has a reputation for relying on people's self-reports, which are considered soft (or not related to anything important) in scientific parlance. Perhaps disclosing deep thoughts and feelings through writing was leading people to overestimate their health in their reports—maybe they felt some emotional connection to the researchers after this powerful disclosure process and were trying to help the researchers out. By examining different types of outcomes, Josh could look at a wider array of objectively measured outcomes such as those measuring immune function.

After combing through the scientific articles and selecting the dozen or so best studies, Josh applied the meta-analytic methods. Several promising findings emerged. Most important, people who wrote about their deepest thoughts and feelings related to stressful or traumatic experiences had reliable improvements in health in the two to three months after writing. Although there were also improvements in people's self-reports of their health, there were equally large effects on people's physiological functioning.

There were some unexpected findings as well. The results of questionnaires that asked about health behaviors—such as healthy eating, exercising, taking medication, and the like—were not influenced by writing. Although some had suggested that writing may be beneficial as a result of better self-care activities, this explanation was not supported by Josh's analysis. Finally, he found that writing reliably but temporarily increased people's feelings of distress. Interestingly, the degree to which people felt distressed was unrelated to subsequent long-term mental or physical health changes. If you were thinking that a "no pain, no gain" explanation could account for the value of writing, it is not that simple. Even though most people felt somewhat distressed by writing, it turns out that suffering more in your writing doesn't lead to more improvements later.

One other observation was critically important: All of the early writing studies relied on people who were physically healthy. If this method is good for people's health, he asked, why haven't any researchers looked at people suffering from chronic disease?

When Josh's meta-analysis was published in the *Journal of Consulting and Clinical Psychology*, in 1998, it had an immediate impact. Researchers around the world realized that there might be something to this expressive writing and began conducting an array of innovative and interesting studies. Within the next several years, a surge of study findings were published that included wildly broad and diverse samples—people with a variety of acute and chronic disease, with major and minor mental health problems. Other studies employed people who were quite healthy but who were trying to master new skills, do better in college, or exhibit greater creativity.

The net effect of Josh's meta-analysis is that it demonstrated the potential value of expressive writing. His paper, however, challenged researchers at the time to explain why it worked. Clearly, when people wrote about emotional upheavals, something important was happening. But what? What precisely happens when people are given the opportunity to disclose their secrets and emotions to others?

Try Expressive Writing

Find a quiet time and place for this next writing exercise. Write for 20 to 30 minutes, focusing on your deepest emotions and thoughts about a stressful or upsetting experience in your life. Whatever you choose to write about, it is critical that you really let go and explore your very deepest emotions and thoughts. Write continuously, and don't worry about spelling, grammar, or style.

Warning: Many people report that after writing, they sometimes feel somewhat sad, although this typically goes away in a couple of hours. If you find that you are getting extremely upset about a writing topic, simply stop writing or change topics.

CHAPTER 3

What's on Your Mind?

HEALTH BENEFITS OF VERBAL AND WRITTEN DISCLOSURE

A therapist recently told the following story of his client, "Barbara":

> "After a late dinner with friends, Barbara got into her car and, after locking the doors, heard the voice of a strange man from the backseat. Holding a knife, he ordered her to drive to a particular city park where, he said, he intended to rape her. As Barbara drove to the park, she started to accelerate. Between sobs, she lied that she had cancer and would soon be dying. Speeding up to 70 mph on the deserted city streets, she noted that she might as well kill them both. As she approached a busy intersection, Barbara warned the man that if he wanted to live, he had better jump out while he could. He jumped from the car as she slowed to make a turn."

The story doesn't end there. Barbara was understandably upset by the event and called her therapist the next morning. When she met with him later that day, he recommended that she tell her story to everyone she met. The more she told the story, he claimed, the more quickly her anxiety symptoms would disappear. Why might talking about a trauma help to cure the trauma? This is intuitively sound advice. But why?

Talking about a trauma is a natural human response. When this need to disclose is blocked or inhibited, stress and illness result. Beyond the potential dangers of long-term inhibition, there is something positive about confronting upsetting experiences. Barbara needed more than the release of inhibition. She needed to come to terms with her terrifying experience. Talking, according to the therapists, was a good way to do this.

Talking about a trauma goes beyond merely moving past inhibition. Usually, when someone talks about a trauma, another person listens. In the case of Barbara, her listeners told her that she was fast thinking, competent, and brave. When she explained that she was still upset, they assured her that her feelings were normal and that they were available to help her in any way. In other cases, talking about a trauma can result in other benefits such as advice, attention, sympathy, financial assistance, and a way of excusing the individuals from carrying out their normal responsibilities.

Although these social benefits can be valuable, there is much more to be gained from talking about upsetting experiences. Specifically, the act of talking can change the ways we think and feel about traumatic events and about ourselves.

The Role of Talking in Achieving Catharsis versus Insight

Most therapists agree that talking about an upsetting experience is psychologically beneficial. The agreement ends there. Some think that talking about a trauma is primarily valuable in achieving catharsis by getting the person to express pent-up emotions. Others believe that talking helps the client attain insight into the causes of the difficulties with the trauma and their potential cures. Others argue other perspectives as to when and why talking may be helpful, and this argument has changed over time as theories and clinical practices have evolved.

In the late 1800s, the young Austrian physician Sigmund Freud began to piece together an overarching theory of personality that pointed to the reasons that confronting a trauma was beneficial. Many of Freud's early ideas stemmed from a technique pioneered by another physician named Josef Breuer, typically called "the talking cure."

In his medical practice, Breuer found that hypnosis was effective in treating people suffering from symptoms such as paralysis, blindness, or deafness that had no apparent physical basis. His most important patient was a 21-year-old woman, referred to as Anna O., who suffered from a variety of problems ranging from a refusal to drink liquids to partial paralysis on the right side of her body. During his sessions with Anna O., Breuer required her to talk while hypnotized about her early experiences with each of her symptoms. For example, one day she talked about her feelings of anger and disgust in seeing a dog drink water from a glass. Immediately after venting her feelings about this episode, Anna O. overcame her refusal to drink liquids. According to Breuer, talking about the causes of symptoms in some way cured them.

Freud was fascinated by Breuer's reports. Although he, too, experimented with hypnosis, Freud believed that he could get comparable results without hypnosis by having his own patients merely talk about their deepest feelings and thoughts while in a relaxed state. Despite such differences in approach, both Freud and Breuer believed that the value of the talking cure lay in its ability to release pent-up feelings that the person was holding back. The two men reasoned that the release of these pent-up feelings, or catharsis, discharged psychic tension in the same way that removing the lid from a pot of boiling water slows the boiling.

Although Freud eventually downplayed the importance of the cathartic method, many of his followers continue to extol its benefits. Unfortunately, the definition of catharsis has evolved to mean the mere venting of emotion rather than the reflective linking of thoughts and feelings. Today, many of the more fringy schools of thought argue that the venting of emotion by screaming, crying, laughing, or other means can permanently improve psychological and physical health. The general scientific consensus now disputes this. A large number of good scientific studies conclude that the mere expression of emotion is usually not beneficial on its own. Rather, people typically must learn to recognize and identify their emotional reactions to events. Talking (and other forms of expression) is beneficial when it helps people make sense of their experiences. We will return to precisely how and why expressive writing might help in more detail in Chapter 9.

The Case of Joey

A change comes over people when they disclose traumatic experiences for the first time. A powerful example can be seen during a stress interview with Joey, a brawny Vietnam veteran who was diagnosed with PTSD. Joey had been referred to a therapist by a county judge after he had physically threatened his boss. After Joey's first session, the therapist brought Joey to one of our labs to evaluate Joey's biological responses during a session. Once in the lab, Joey appeared relatively calm and answered the therapist's initial questions in a matter-of-fact way.

During the first 20 minutes of the interview, Joey talked about his childhood, his current living situation, and several of his experiences in Vietnam. Joey's physiological levels changed radically when he briefly remarked about one of the jungle outposts where he had been stationed. The therapist in charge pressed Joey for more details about the outpost. All of a sudden, Joey's entire demeanor changed. His voice dropped and he started to speak in a low, rapid monotone. He began a story about going out on a routine patrol with his buddy. They were about a mile from the base camp when his life changed.

> There was a burst of gunfire and my buddy fell to the ground, half of his head blown off. I looked up and a [North Vietnamese soldier] was running into a shed carrying a machine gun. I ran to the shed, jumped through the door and fired, hitting them in both legs. It was a woman who had shot my buddy and who was bleeding on the ground. We stared into each other's eyes. I ripped off her clothes and made love to her. Before I knew it, I could hear choppers overhead—ours. I pulled out my knife and slit her throat. I loved her. I killed her.

It had been 15 years since this had happened, and Joey had never told anyone. The therapist was in a state of shock but continued to explore Joey's thoughts and feelings about this horror. After about 40 minutes of calmly talking about the incident, Joey began to cry. Soon thereafter, the veil lifted and Joey returned to his normal speaking voice. By the end of the session, Joey was fatigued and his physiological levels indicated that he was relatively relaxed. In commenting on his experience in the laboratory, Joey admitted surprise at his revealing what had happened in Vietnam: "It felt like another person was describing my thoughts."

The Letting-Go Experience

The change that came over Joey is surprisingly common. Often, when people in our experiments either talk or write about deeply personal secrets, certain aspects of their personalities temporarily change. This change is part of a "letting-go" experience in that the usual inhibitions are no longer in force. During the time that people are letting go, profound changes often occur in their speech and writing styles as well as their physiological levels. The letting-go experience is closely linked to a variety of altered states of consciousness, such as a trance-like state in psychotherapy. Basically, any technique that induces a state of relaxation while maintaining mental alertness will promote the letting-go experience.

In several of our experiments, people have been asked to talk into tape recorders about their most traumatic experiences as well as superficial topics. Those individuals who have disclosed particularly intimate sides of themselves have shown a variety of changes in their voice and speaking style. For example, a woman who participated in the very first experiment of this kind initially described her plans for the day in a singsongy, high-pitched, almost childlike way. A few minutes later, as she described stealing $100 from an open cash register, both the volume and pitch of her voice were lower. The voice characteristics were so different that the two recordings sounded as though they were made by different women.

A second reliable effect concerns speaking rate. The more traumatic the topic, the faster people talk. In fact, those participants who reported never having told anyone about their traumas were the ones who tended to speak the most rapidly. The experiment had provided the opportunity for many of these people to talk about events that they clearly had thought about for months or even years. The floodgates were open, and the words poured out.

The letting-go experience is just as obvious when participants write as when they talk about upsetting events. As with talking, people write faster when disclosing traumas than when describing superficial objects or events. More striking, however, are changes in handwriting. Often, handwriting switches from block to cursive and back to block lettering within the same essay as the writers switch from one topic to another. Similar changes can be seen in the slant of the letters, pen pressure, cross-outs, and general neatness as a function of topic.

Another intriguing phenomenon concerns how people talk and write about upsetting and personal experiences. For example, two conflicting topics often activate one another—apparently without the person's awareness. When one topic is introduced, its opposite soon follows. Here are some examples from one of the writing studies.

A 20-year-old college junior writes:

> *I love my parents. We have a perfect family life. My parents support me in whatever I do. I wouldn't change anything about my childhood, really. . . . [Later in the same essay] My father has been such a bastard, I know that he has something going with his secretary. My mother takes it out on me. I have to wear the clothes she wants, date the boys she wants.*

This pattern is quite common. In fact, whenever an essay begins with something like "we have such a close family" or "my little sister is *so* great," 9 times out of 10, the discloser soon changes tone and eventually unleashes a verbal attack on his or her family, sister, or whomever. As an aside, a particularly revealing word is *really*—as in "I respect my roommate, really." Translated, this means "I don't respect my roommate." Usually the word appears toward the beginning of an essay when the writer is still holding back. In fact, words like *really* (or *honestly* and *truly*) often indicate inhibition. Once writers move into the letting-go mode, these words rarely appear.

A different example of an issue emerging from an emotionally powerful topic can be seen in an 18-year-old freshman who, once he remembered that his mother held his spelling in low regard, temporarily lost his spelling skills:

> *Today, my mother sent a care package and I was very excited until I opened it. It was all old things that I had left in my room, bills, old letters, etc. I began to realize that my past could follow me anywhere. My mother sent me an old book I used to have on commonly mispelled words. It allmost ofended me. That was such a reminder of all the old habbits and imature actions I felt like a child again.*

Finally, the sequence of topics that people disclose is often meaningful. For example, a married woman who was attracted to someone besides her spouse showed a similar transition in topics during each day of the experiment:

> *I deeply care about Robert, but know that we can never get involved. Sam [her husband] is working on a new project that could mean a lot of money for us. . . .*

[As a teenager] I looked up to football players like Robert, even though I was afraid to date them. I feel bad that I have criticized Sam and his obsession with tennis. Robert thinks the reason I quit college was to anger my folks. Sam graduated with honors. . . .

Topic cueing usually goes in only one direction. That is, topic A (in this case, Robert) is always followed by topic B (Sam), rarely vice versa. Further, topic cueing, changes in writing style, and less use of words like *really* are most apparent when people are no longer inhibiting.

The letting-go experience is similar to a trance state. Many people report losing their sense of time and place while disclosing their intimate secrets. Some clinicians, such as Milton Erickson, consider the letting-go experience a form of hypnotic state. Indeed, Erickson asserts that this psychological state is therapeutically valuable in both learning about the client's underlying problems and influencing the direction of therapy. As we have found, once people are in this hypnotic state, they are no longer self-conscious, worried about pleasing others, or concerned about their normal daily hassles. The letting-go experience signals the temporary stripping away of many of our normal social constraints or inhibitions.

The Physiology of Inhibition and Confession: Heavy Heart, Sweaty Hands

The letting-go experience sounds magical, even mystical. During the time that people were in this letting-go state, a number of remarkable physiological changes occurred. To appreciate them, consider how our bodies react when we are threatened.

Our bodies have evolved to respond almost immediately to stressors—anything we perceive in our environment that we think has the potential to threaten or harm us. If someone yells "Fire!" or if we see a rabid dog about to pounce on us, we need to be able to think and behave quickly. We usually can do this thanks to the action of the autonomic nervous system. The autonomic nervous system controls our blood pressure, breathing rate, and dozens of other automatic physiological/biological functions needed in times of emergency. In short, the autonomic nervous system controls the fight-or-flight reaction.

One of the long-standing debates among psychophysiologists (a fancy title for those who study the interplay of psychological or emotional states with biological and physiological processes in the body) concerns the reaction of the nervous system to different stressors. That is, are there different biological patterns to different types of stressors? Or does the autonomic nervous system just fire generally to any kind of stress? The emerging consensus is that both are likely correct to a degree—there are general response patterns, but the autonomic nervous system also may tailor its response to different stressful situations.

There is good evidence that the body responds differently to situations where the people must inhibit their behaviors versus when they must be behaviorally active. Various physiological indicators help us understand these processes. We can see markers of physiological inhibition by increases in how much our hands perspire—which we can measure using skin conductance (formerly called GSR, for galvanic skin response). Physiological activation, on the other hand, can be seen through changes in the cardiovascular system such as increases in heart rate.

By getting independent physiological measures of inhibition and activation, we can learn the degree to which confession is, in fact, a clear release of inhibitions. Further, we now have a basis for evaluating the letting-go experience.

The Body's Response to Confession

Why are we telling you all of this? Because of Latoya, a former student and good friend who dropped by Jamie's office one day. Since it was almost noon, he suggested that they go across the street for a sandwich. As soon as they sat down, it was clear something was the matter. Latoya wasn't hungry, and when asked why, she began to cry. It was the first anniversary of the death of both of her parents, who had been killed in a private plane accident. Latoya was miserable, and lunch was ruined. "Let's go back to my office and talk about it," Jamie suggested. As they walked back, she discussed her parents. Then it hit him. "How would you feel about going to the lab and talking about your parents while you are hooked up?"

Fortunately, Latoya was well acquainted with his eccentricities and agreed to be "hooked up" to his skin conductance apparatus. Over the course of the interview, Latoya talked about the details of the accident, including going to the morgue to identify her parents' bodies. Jamie also asked her to discuss some relatively trivial topics, such as her plans for the remainder of the day. At other times, Latoya was asked to stop talking and merely to think about the deaths and about more trivial issues. This was an emotionally wrenching experience for both of them. When talking and thinking about her parents' deaths, Latoya was clearly in great pain. In addition to crying occasionally, she would sometimes get into a reverie as though she were reliving that horrible day.

Latoya's physiological reactions were fascinating. Whenever she talked or thought about the deaths, her skin conductance levels dropped dramatically. Talking and thinking about superficial topics, on the other hand, was associated with increases in skin conductance. Letting go and confronting the deaths, then, represented a reduction in inhibition. In this particular setting, whenever Latoya was instructed to think or talk about trivial topics, her skin conductance increased— presumably because she was actively blocking out or inhibiting her feelings and thoughts about the deaths.

The case of Latoya was important for several reasons. Above all, it appeared as though skin conductance was a potential measure of the letting-go experience. In addition, her data hinted that confronting traumatic experiences was, in fact, indicative of a reduction of inhibition. Unfortunately, case studies are often intoxicating but misleading. Just because Latoya's body worked in a theoretically meaningful way was no assurance that others' bodies did likewise. A controlled experiment was needed.

High Disclosers versus Low Disclosers

Jamie, along with two of his students, Cherie Hughes and Robin O'Heeron, conducted two similar experiments. The gist of the studies was that students were asked to talk about two different topics for about 5 minutes each: the most traumatic experiences of their lives and their plans for the remainder of the day. While they talked into a tape recorder, their skin conductance, blood pressure, heart rate, facial muscle tension, and hand temperature were continuously measured. The night before the experiment, each participant was called and told all about the study. It was important that they had thought about what they would say in the experiment.

Consider this study from the volunteer's perspective. You are called by a perfect stranger who identifies herself as a graduate student in psychology. You are told that if you choose to participate, you will talk into a tape recorder about the most traumatic, personal, upsetting event of your life while attached to numerous wires and tubes measuring your reactions. During the time that you talk, you will be alone in a quiet and dimly lit room in the basement of the psychology department. You are assured, of course, that everything you say will be kept strictly confidential.

There was some doubt that people would divulge their deepest secrets in such a short amount of time, under such unusual circumstances. Those doubts were erased as soon as the first people came to the lab. In the two experiments, roughly a quarter of the participants cried when disclosing their traumatic experiences. The choice of topics, the self-ratings the volunteers made about their own disclosures, and our own evaluations of the tape recordings indicated that this technique was quite powerful. Ironically, the power of the first experiment wasn't apparent until it was completed. Although Jamie's research team had assumed that the participants talked about traumas for a full five minutes, their timer was malfunctioning. They actually had talked for only about three and a half minutes.

In listening to the tape recordings of people talking about traumas in this early work, people seemed to fall into two categories: those who disclosed a great deal and those who seemed to be holding back. The high disclosers, who represented about half of the participants, were those who evidenced signs of the letting-go experience, including change in voice, displays of emotion, and their revealing highly personal sides of themselves. Low disclosers, on the other hand, were much less involved in what they said. Although the low disclosers often talked about extremely traumatic events, at least superficially, they seemed to hold back their feelings much more than the high disclosers. In fact, a group of independent judges who listened to each of the tapes had little difficulty in distinguishing high from low disclosers.

In looking at the physiological data, the high disclosers behaved similarly to Latoya. As a group, for example, high disclosers had lower skin conductance levels when talking about traumatic experiences than when discussing their plans for the day. In addition to the skin conductance findings, the high disclosers exhibited an intriguing pattern of blood pressure and heart rate responses. Overall, their blood pressure and heart rate levels were highest during the time they talked about traumas. This makes sense from an activation perspective, since almost half of the high disclosers cried—which tends to involve movement in much of the body. More interestingly, however, these people showed lower blood pressures *after* confessing than before the experiment started.

Compared with the high disclosers, the low disclosers did not seem to get emotionally involved with the study. None cried; most admitted what they talked about was only moderately personal or emotional. Their biological signals reflected this lack of involvement. The only reliable effect across the two studies was that their skin conductance levels were higher when they tried to confront traumas than when they talked about their plans for the day. For the low disclosers, then, broaching personal topics required physiological work. That is, they had to hold back important emotions and thoughts when talking about their traumas.

When (and if) people really let go and disclose their very deepest thoughts and feelings, a number of immediate and long-term bodily changes occur. Skin conductance, an indicator of inhibition, drops during the confession (i.e., when there is no longer the effort associated with active inhibition). Blood pressure, heart rate, and other cardiovascular changes increase during the confession. After high disclosers confide, however, their blood pressures drop to levels below what they had been when they entered the study.

Do these results mean if you really let go and disclose your most traumatic experiences that your blood pressure will permanently drop to low levels and that your hands will never sweat again? Yes . . . *really*. (Translation: Of course not.) First of all, these early studies were done with generally healthy college students, not grizzled, hypertensive, harried adults. Also the blood pressure drops were statistically reliable, but the reductions were not medically significant (about 6 mm Hg for both systolic and diastolic blood pressure).

Finally, these results were most reliable for the high disclosers. We still can't fully explain why the other half of our participants didn't exhibit the letting-go experience. One very real possibility is that low disclosers didn't trust us and were not about to reveal their deepest secrets to a group of strangers in the dingy basement of the psychology building. Alternatively, some of the low disclosers might not have the ability to let go for reasons we simply could not discern at the time.

Since this early work, several studies have been conducted exploring a wide range of physiological processes. For example, Kimberly McGuire and her colleagues looked at people with high blood pressure. Some participants were asked to write about emotional topics and others to write about everyday nonemotional experiences. Blood pressure dropped drastically in the expressive writing group, and these changes were not observed among those who wrote about nonemotional topics. A similar pattern was found by a team in the United Kingdom among people who had recently experienced a heart attack, or myocardial infarction. Those who wrote about their thoughts and feelings related to their heart attacks showed a decrease in prescribed medications, fewer reported cardiac symptoms, and lower diastolic blood pressure five months after the disclosure intervention was over.

Writing to Disclose or Confess

Find a quiet time and place for this next writing exercise. Think of a topic that you have not previously discussed or disclosed with others; perhaps you have even inhibited talking or thinking about it. Write about this topic for 20 to 30 minutes; as in prior exercises, try to write continuously and do not worry about style, spelling, and so forth.

When done, reflect on how you felt physiologically—how did you feel during writing? After writing? Review your writing: Do you notice any patterns or insights to be gained? You might repeat this exercise over several days and see if additional changes or insights.

This Is Your Brain on Confession

Confronting traumas has some powerful effects on the body. In the early years of this work, we had seen how disclosing secrets had beneficially affected immune function, blood pressure, heart rate, and skin conductance, and reduced physician visits for illness. Since then, research from labs around the world revealed how disclosure through expressive writing or talking affected a much larger array of biological systems and illnesses.

All of these bodily changes are merely reflections of something happening in the brain. What is the brain doing when a person lets go and discloses upsetting experiences? Could it be measured? If so, would the findings be meaningful?

Think back to the case of Joey, the Vietnam veteran. Before participating in the interview, he had recurring images, thoughts, and emotions about raping and killing the woman in Vietnam. By his own admission, he also recalled conflicting and powerful feelings of respect and even love for the woman, as well as anger about her killing his buddy. On top of all of this, in his own mind he had to be on guard against telling others about this experience. Clearly, these issues were not well integrated. As this line of thinking goes, different parts of this complex experience were probably being processed independently in different parts of his brain. However, because he did not allow himself to bring these different parts of the same experience together, he never resolved the issues.

Advances in neuroscience since the original publication of this book have been astounding. Early on, both Josh and Jamie had speculated about possible brain-related changes that could possibly explain the benefits of expressive writing. Now, however, researchers have new ways to study the inner workings of the human brain while people are dealing with emotional topics. You have likely heard of fMRI—functional magnetic resonance imaging. Methods such as fMRI allow us to see inside your brain by looking at what parts are active when performing some cognitive or emotional task or when thinking about particular topics.

Although there are many labs conducting this kind of work, some exceptional work has been done by Matthew Lieberman and his colleagues at UCLA. Lieberman's group reports that people who were deathly afraid of spiders and expressed those fears when exposed to a real spider were able to physically move closer to the spider than those who merely looked at the spider. Putting those fears into language appeared to confer some protective benefit. Lieberman broadly refers to this process as affect labeling—putting negative emotions into words seems to blunt their effect on us. But how might this occur? They have found that there is a part of the brain, the right prefrontal cortex, involved in effortful control over our emotional states. When this part of the brain "turns on," other parts of the brain that are related to strong negative emotions—such as the amygdala—are turned off. In other words, putting our deeply emotional experiences into language and words facilitates our brain's capacity to help us manage our emotional states.

The Laboratory's Role in Confession

By now it should be clear that people readily disclose their deepest secrets once they are in the psychology laboratory. Even when they are recorded, when sensors and cuffs are attached to their arms, hands, and faces, or their blood is drawn, participants let go and reveal the most intimate sides of themselves. If you were in one of these studies, would you show signs of the letting-go experience?

We have asked ourselves that question many times. A laboratory experiment is a unique event. The participant is put in a situation where he or she can divulge anything without repercussion. In many ways, it is safer than talking to a close friend, entering psychotherapy, or, for many people, praying. In the laboratory, we have inadvertently provided people with a safe, nonjudgmental haven for disclosure.

Interestingly, these experiments say a great deal about both the power of the laboratory and the nature of confession. The context of the laboratory signals that the participants do not need to inhibit their thoughts and feelings the way they usually do. The underlying message that we try to convey is "say whatever you want . . . it doesn't matter to us . . . we are simply a group of researchers interested in what makes you tick."

Although the laboratory provides a safe setting to disclose secrets, the degree to which participants readily do so is also important. People seem to have an underlying urge to confess. Although many have been holding back their personal secrets for months or years, they are still eager to discuss them when provided the right opportunity to do so. Whether there is a true biological need to confess is certainly debatable. In any case, people are open to disclosing aspects of themselves or their behavior that are potentially humiliating, shameful, or downright illegal. Why would people be willing to do this? One explanation comes from recent work by Brené Brown (2010; 2012), in which she compellingly argues that embracing these feelings, broadly subsumed under a willingness to accept and be open to our own vulnerability, is at the core of overcoming shame and fear. Doing so allows us to live more authentic lives and forge more wholehearted and sustaining connections with others. We will return to these and related themes throughout the book.

The physiological results that have been summarized (and many more not included) point to the profound power of confession. Or, perhaps, the profound effort involved in inhibition. It is not merely expressing thoughts and feelings, but also confessing, that has potent and measurable effects on our biology. When disclosing deeply personal experiences, there are immediate changes in brain activation, skin conductance levels, and overt behavioral correlates of the letting-go experience. After confessions, significant drops in blood pressure and heart rate as well as improvements in immune function occur. In the weeks and months afterward, people's physical and psychological health is improved.

CHAPTER 4

Dealing with Chronic Health Problems Using Expressive Writing

The story of the expressive writing technique is a case study in the sociology of science. The first writing study piqued the interest of several researchers. Some were excited about the potential usefulness of the method, and others were skeptical about whether it was even valid. In the decade after the first publication in 1986, over a dozen studies were published that indicated that the effects were real. Almost all of the studies were conducted with healthy college students.

Healthy college students? Is this really the best group of people from whom to learn whether expressive writing can influence physical and mental health? If writing truly has broad value, it should boost the health of people who are suffering from real diseases. Yes, expressive writing was associated with lower rates of upper respiratory infections among 18-year-old college students, but what about major debilitating and even life-threatening diseases that plague all cultures?

Fortunately, the college student projects had helped to answer some central questions. Expressive writing influenced physician visits over several months—that is, the effects were not so transient that they evaporated within minutes or hours after an experiment. The responses to writing were also affecting basic biological processes. Writing affected the immune system, the autonomic nervous system (including heart rate, blood pressure, and skin conductance), social factors, and even sleep patterns. Plus, there was some promising evidence that it influenced the ways students felt emotionally. In other words, there were compelling reasons to think that expressive writing *could* influence the course of chronic diseases.

Beginning Research on Chronic Conditions and Expressive Writing

While Jamie was thinking of doing a large-scale study on people with chronic diseases, Josh had already started doing one. Working with a group of colleagues at Stony Brook University's medical school, Josh recruited medical patients with chronic asthma or rheumatoid arthritis who had all been assessed by physicians. For the asthma patients, their lung function was examined; for those with arthritis, their joint stiffness and range of movement were assessed. Half the patients were assigned to write about the most stressful or traumatic experiences of their lives, and the other half were asked to write about daily plans. Patients' health and disease status was reexamined several times, up to four months after writing.

The results were astonishing. Patients who wrote about emotional upheavals had objective improvements in lung function (those with asthma) and joint health (patients with arthritis) compared to those who wrote about control topics. The size of the improvements was impressive as well—the majority of patients reported meaningful improvements in quality of life similar to benefits that would be expected by a successful new drug treatment.

Josh's subsequent paper in the *Journal of the American Medical Association*, or *JAMA*, made big news. It suggested that expressive writing might be a useful addition to medical care in the treatment of patients. In other words, people suffering from major chronic disease could get meaningful improvements in their disease by disclosing their deepest thoughts and feelings. His study also energized the expressive writing research community. If writing could influence the lives of people with arthritis and asthma, what about other diseases such as cancer, heart disease, or HIV? Discussions among psychological researchers interested in writing became a bit heady and self-important—we thought we had a tool that could cure the ills of the world. Was there no limit to the value of writing?

It turns out there was. Perhaps the biggest limitation was in our conceptualization of disease itself.

The Nature of Diseases: A Side Note
on Psychosomatics

In the wake of Sigmund Freud's early papers on psychoanalysis and mental illness, a number of his followers suggested that physical health could also be influenced by psychological or emotional states. By the 1950s, the field of psychosomatics was an accepted area of study at most medical schools. The underlying idea was that psychological conflict could be expressed through physiological changes or even manifest as illnesses. Some argued that asthma was the result of a smothering mother. Skin problems reflected the psychological state of being picked on by others.

More careful and controlled research subsequently failed to support many of the specific Freudian assumptions, and by the 1980s virtually no Freudian influence existed in either medical schools or psychology departments. Since then, a more palatable and scientifically supported version of the psychosomatic view has emerged. At its simplest, when people are in some way stressed or in conflict, clear and measurable biological changes can occur. Further, these short-term biological changes, if they occur over extended periods of time, can influence or exacerbate diseases. In contrast to the old Freudian perspective, most modern psychosomatic theorists don't make specific predictions about which disease a person is likely to get in response to particular types of stress or conflict. Rather, the idea is that stress or conflict will likely wear down a range of bodily systems, and symptoms or illness will emerge in the systems that are most vulnerable. One person might be prone to diabetes, another to heart disease, and yet a third to digestive problems. On top of that, the habits people adopt will have a powerful influence on stress-related illness patterns. Smokers are more likely to have heart and lung problems; people who drink too much alcohol may be prone to liver ailments.

Sadly, diseases are not as straightforward as you might think. Imagine you are walking barefoot and get a splinter in your foot. It hurts a bit, and you can't pull it out because it is so small. Within an hour, you have found some tweezers and a good light and begin the ordeal of removing it. You will likely notice three biological changes: swelling, increased heat at the site of the swelling, and pain when you apply pressure to the swollen area. You probably are thinking that the pain and inflammation are caused by the splinter. Not so fast.

If we get a bit technical, and also oversimplify a little, the symptoms you are experiencing are your body's reaction to the damage caused by the splinter and to the bacteria on the splinter. The splinter may have had a small number of relatively benign bacteria, but your immune system reacted aggressively. Tens of thousands of white blood cells converged on the splinter, causing inflammation and generating heat. These actions reduced circulation around the splinter, lowering the likelihood that any bacteria would get into the bloodstream. The heat would also help kill any sensitive bacteria. The increased pain will motivate you to not put pressure on the area. Walking or poking the area could reduce the swelling and allow the spread of bacteria.

Here's the irony: You might think that the problem is the swelling, heat, and pain. But those are your body's solutions to the real problem—the possible spread of dangerous bacteria or other toxins. The splinter and bacteria on their own in most cases wouldn't cause you any harm. Because you have an active and healthy immune system, your body is just being vigilant.

Think back to the first writing studies dealing with reduced physician visits. Most of the student health center visits dealt with upper respiratory infections—usually simple colds or flu. A cold is an infection caused by a virus that typically results in inflammation, a running and stuffy nose, and a sore throat. Like our body's reaction to a splinter, what we think is the disease is really our body's reaction to a relatively benign virus.

The reason we get these symptoms in response to the cold virus is that our immune system is working efficiently. At other times, however, our immune systems can be suppressed. High levels of stress, for example, can temporarily block parts of the immune response. Steroid drugs such as cortisone can do the same. When this happens, bacteria and viruses in the body can reproduce and spread alarmingly. Once the stress is over or we stop taking cortisone, our immune systems start working at full force. This can mean major inflammation, pain, and high body temperature. Once again, then, the symptoms of the cold are really your body's attempt at the cure.

An interesting side note. If you are like most people, you may have gotten sick immediately after a major life stressor ended: after a difficult semester in college, immediately after you got married, or once you'd finished a particularly important project. If it makes you feel any better, your illness was really just your body telling you that it needed to kill off a number of bugs that it hadn't been able to during the time you were highly stressed and needed to get other important jobs done.

The Biology and Psychology of Expressive Writing

Why does expressive writing improve health? Earlier, we glibly implied that it enhanced immune activity. This is only partially true. Sometimes, illness is the immune response itself. In fact, some diseases such as arthritis, asthma, AIDS, some features of cancer, and possibly even depression, may reflect alterations or malfunctioning of the immune system.

After several decades of expressive writing studies, the scientific community is beginning to get a broader appreciation of the reasons writing can be helpful. All chronic diseases have at least three broad components that influence the course of illness: their biological underpinnings, social and emotional factors related to the disease, and ways that people's behaviors can prevent, reduce, or worsen the course of the disease.

THE BIOLOGICAL MECHANISMS OF DISEASE

There are several ways that expressive writing could influence disease processes directly. Individuals who are under a great deal of stress typically have higher levels of stress hormones in their system than people not under stress. Two of the most common stress hormones are cortisol and epinephrine (also called adrenaline). There is considerable evidence that cortisol suppresses immune activity and that adrenaline increases blood pressure and can even affect the digestive system. Both have been implicated in sleep disruption as well.

To date, the most likely way that expressive writing could improve health would be through the reduction of long-term stress. If writing helped people resolve major conflicts, their sleep would likely improve, their stress levels would return to more normal levels, and their immune systems could start working more efficiently.

Would these biological changes influence, say, our reaction to the splinter? Actually, yes. In the last decade there have been several studies exploring writing and wound healing. The studies are quite compelling—the general approach is that volunteers come into a laboratory and agree to have a small punch biopsy, typically on their arm. This involves, if you haven't had one before, a sterile device that takes out a small chunk of flesh. A by-product of this procedure is that it produces a small, consistent wound that will typically heal over a couple of weeks. Researchers then use a high-resolution ultrasound scanner or similar technology to track wound healing. This provides a perfect opportunity to see what effect expressive writing may have on the healing process in wounds. John Weinman and his colleagues at King's College London used this approach with healthy volunteers who were asked to write about emotional upheavals or control topics after the experimental wound. The findings were clear. The wounds healed much faster among the people asked to write about emotional topics. Another study from the New Zealand lab of Liz Broadbent at the University of Auckland School of Medicine, who studied older adults, found similar effects—those completing expressive writing showed much faster rates of healing than those writing about neutral topics.

What about improvements that might have occurred in Josh's study with people suffering from rheumatoid arthritis or asthma? This is more difficult to answer. He did find objective improvements in joint movement and lung function measures up to four months afterward. But he didn't have any evidence for changes in cortisol or immune markers, and he didn't see major changes in behavior. Something clearly changed among those who had participated in the expressive writing condition, but it appeared to be something that was not measured.

As we begin looking at increasingly complex diseases that may persist for years, the underlying biology of both the disease and the healing processes becomes too complex to disentangle—at least for the time being. One thing that is safe to assume is that expressive writing does *not* kill cancer cells or viruses associated with serious illness such as AIDS. It can clearly help boost immune function to a certain degree, but it is not a panacea and should not replace appropriate medical care.

SOCIAL AND EMOTIONAL CONTRIBUTORS TO DISEASE

Chronic disease is more than the pathogens and reactions of the immune system. Diseases also change the ways people think and look at their worlds. Think back to the splinter example. If you get a splinter as you are putting on your wedding dress two minutes before you go down the aisle, you probably won't notice the splinter, and even if you do, it will be out of your mind quickly. Sometimes symptoms and health problems cause us to worry and lose sleep, and skyrocket our anxiety levels; other times, the same health problems hardly register.

Some health conditions are so psychologically or socially threatening that if our friends knew about them, we might be shamed or outright rejected by them. Think of the unmarried Hester Prynne getting pregnant in Nathaniel Hawthorne's *The Scarlet Letter*. Or a young gay man in the 1980s diagnosed with AIDS and no one in his family knowing about his sexual orientation. Or the single 55-year-old man who has prostate cancer but doesn't want his friends or prospective love interests to know. All of these examples harken back to the problem of secrets. Not only are the people dealing with an unwanted pregnancy or a life-threatening disease; they are also having to contend with a giant secret that dominates their thoughts, feelings, and social behaviors.

There is a long history of research showing that paying attention to pain and other physical symptoms often makes them worse. If you have just been diagnosed with cancer, you will immediately begin paying attention to every symptom you experience. Should you decide to keep the diagnosis secret, you will likely avoid talking with close friends and, instead, spend more time alone concentrating on your body. This pattern heightens feelings of anxiety, fear, and possibly anger. Two people who have exactly the same biological states could have completely different experiences. One who is alone and obsessing about his health will feel and act sicker than the other who is open and talking with her friends.

You can probably see how expressive writing can influence people's perceptions of their own health. Coming to terms with emotional upheavals and even concerns about health problems will help people stop ruminating about their fears and problems. (And, in turn, the less they are worried about their health, the less likely they will be to run to the doctor or take unneeded medication—raising other explanations we turn to below.) In some cases, expressive writing may not directly influence biological processes at all but rather shake people out of a cycle of secrecy and worrying about their health.

SELF-CARE AND DISEASE MANAGEMENT

Expressive writing can also influence health by changing the ways people behave in the face of their disease. The general medical wisdom is that the prevention and treatment of disease can be helped if people exercise, eat wisely, take the right medications at the right time, and don't smoke or otherwise abuse their bodies.

It's possible, then, that expressive writing could influence people's health through an indirect route of helping people live healthier lifestyles. There have been at least two studies suggesting that expressive writing can help people stop smoking and several others showing improved sleep following writing. Most experiments, however, that have simply had people write about traumatic experiences and have found improved general health have not reported many changes in their health-relevant behaviors.

Standing back, it should be clearer why it is often difficult to identify how, when, and why expressive writing can influence the health of people suffering from chronic diseases—much less a splinter. In some cases, writing may directly affect the underlying biological processes. In others, writing may bring benefits by simply changing people's emotional states or relationships with others. And finally, writing could be bringing about changes in health styles or health behaviors.

In reality, all three processes—biology, emotional state, and health-related behaviors—interact together. Our biological processes are influenced by changes in moods and our connections with our friends as well as our health-related behaviors. When there are meaningful changes in the course of our disease or biological processes more generally, changes in our moods and behaviors may follow. The interdependence of these processes can lead to downward spirals (when bad things start to feed into one another and things worsen) or virtuous cycles (where some positive changes lead to others and things improve).

Understanding Your Stress

Find a quiet place to try this writing exercise. Start by writing "Stress" at the top of the page; then, under it, write whatever associated word or topic enters your mind. Continue to do this, immediately writing one word or phrase after another as they enter your mind. Don't think too hard, and don't evaluate, censor, or otherwise limit what you associate with each successive word. Keep writing until no more words or topics appear in your mind.

Take a short break and then review your writing. Look at the list of words, topics, and phrases to see if you notice patterns. Are there themes or topics that emerge? Are there patterns in the emotions or meanings of the words? Such patterns may help you understand the nature and impact of stress in your life.

Writing for People with Chronic Disease

There is a very good chance that you or someone close to you will be diagnosed with a major chronic disease in your lifetime. If you are over the age of 50, there is a good chance that you are already living with one. Medical advances have now made it possible for people to live many years, even decades, with chronic diseases while maintaining a good quality of life. The beauty of expressive writing is that it may be helpful above what you are doing now.

Over the last 25 years, there have been a surprising number of writing studies dealing with several chronic health conditions. The studies have varied in quality, the measures used, and the pattern of results. In the pages that follow, we will try to give you brief, simplified summaries of the research on expressive writing and these illnesses, and our best guesses about conditions for which writing may provide benefits and when or where it might not. It will likely be another decade before solid answers are available about the effectiveness of writing for most conditions. This discussion is just a start.

AUTOIMMUNE AND INFLAMMATORY DISORDERS

Our immune systems defend the body from foreign invaders (germs, viruses, etc.). One of the essential features of the immune system is the ability to tell the difference between you and, well, not you. This is not as easy as it sounds. Autoimmune diseases are conditions in which the body's immune system mistakes some of the body's healthy tissues or organs for foreign invaders. Other types of autoimmune diseases, such as asthma, involve the body's immune system mounting particularly aggressive attacks against harmless substances, such as pollen. When this happens, the immune response can be so strong that it places the person's body—and sometimes life itself—at risk. The underlying cause of autoimmune diseases is not well understood. A great deal of recent research is beginning to implicate genes and heredity. Our immune, and inflammatory, processes work very differently in different diseases.

Asthma

In asthma, exaggerated inflammatory processes in the primary airways of the lungs lead to periodic obstruction and difficulties breathing, as well as coughing and wheezing. Approximately 8 percent of the population of the United States suffers from asthma, and almost a quarter of cases are in children. Although many people outgrow it, people can have asthma attacks at unpredictable times—sometimes during periods of high stress or when confronted with a particular trigger such as pollen. Asthma itself is stressful because of its unpredictability and the anxiety it provokes in sufferers undergoing an attack.

To date, there have been a few high-quality studies on expressive writing and asthma. The first, discussed earlier, was by Josh. A more recent study, published in 2015 by Helen Smith and her colleagues in Great Britain, studied asthma patients who attended primary treatment centers. Half were asked to write about emotional upheavals and the remainder about superficial topics. Patients with moderately severe cases of asthma evidenced clear improvements. However, those with mild or with very severe cases did not show benefits.

In other words, if you were not very sick at all, expressive writing did not help—perhaps there was no room to get better. Those who were more seriously ill also didn't benefit—perhaps, here, expressive writing was not potent enough to help. Benefit was observed when patients were moderately impaired by their illness; this might be the sweet spot for expressive writing—where there is room for improvement, but things aren't so bad that more substantial treatment is necessary.

Rheumatoid Arthritis and Other Pain-Related Disorders

Rheumatoid arthritis is a type of arthritis that causes autoimmune and inflammatory processes resulting in swelling, stiffness, and painful areas (often focused in joints), frequently making movement difficult. Although it generally strikes in middle age, some contract it as early as childhood. Women are more likely to be diagnosed with it than men. Generally, once a diagnosis of arthritis has been made, it tends to worsen over time.

Since Josh's original study, there have been others showing that expressive writing can reduce the debilitating symptoms of rheumatoid arthritis and other chronic pain conditions. Patients with either arthritis or lupus were studied by Sharon Danoff-Burg and her colleagues at the University of Albany. She found that those asked to write expressively reported less fatigue three months later. Another study by Mark Lumley and colleagues tested both expressive writing and a cognitive-behavioral skills training intervention to help patients with arthritis. He found that expressive writing produced some initial benefit for the patients, reducing pain and disability, but the benefits dissipated several months after the writing had concluded.

Fibromyalgia is a related condition characterized by persistent musculoskeletal pain, fatigue, and physical sensitivity. Studies examining the use of expressive writing techniques on patients with fibromyalgia have found some evidence that writing can help reduce symptoms and enhance quality of life. For example, expressive writing can produce reductions in pain, fatigue, and restlessness in patients suffering from persistent fibromyalgia. A study out of Stony Brook University found that fibromyalgia patients who were dealing with social stressors benefited from expressive writing. A later study by Hsu and colleagues extended this work, testing the combination of expressive writing coupled with emotional awareness exercises—this combination led to significant pain reduction, better physical function, and reduced tenderness up to six months later in fibromyalgia patients.

Irritable Bowel Syndrome

There are many diseases that influence the function of the gut or, more formally, the gastrointestinal (or GI) system—the stomach, small intestine, colon, and so forth. As you might guess, our guts are very sensitive to emotional and psychological states. In fact, recent evidence has shown that the same neurochemicals that function in our brains, as well as many drugs that target both physical and mental conditions, are also processed in our guts and can influence the function of the GI system.

In theory, expressive writing should have an influence on GI diseases—particularly the chronic conditions known to be sensitive to stress (colitis, Crohn's disease, and many others). Although work in this area is still emerging, early results are very promising. One study examined the use of expressive writing in patients with irritable bowel syndrome, or IBS. IBS is characterized by chronic, but highly variable, abdominal pain, bloating, and alteration of bowel movements (including diarrhea, constipation, or both). Some patients with IBS wrote about their deepest thoughts, feelings, and beliefs regarding the disease and how it was affecting them, and they were compared to other patients who did not write. The writing group showed substantial improvement several months later—notably, the severity of IBS symptoms was reduced at one month and three months after writing, relative to those not writing. Patients who wrote also showed improvements in how they thought about their illness three months later.

HIV/AIDS

HIV (human immunodeficiency virus) is an infectious virus that attacks the immune system, particularly damaging a subset of white blood cells (CD4 cells). These white blood cells are an important part of how the immune system protects against foreign invaders. If HIV progresses, particularly to acquired immunodeficiency syndrome (or AIDS), the impairment in the immune system's capacity to protect against infection can prove deadly.

Several teams of researchers have examined disclosure more generally, and expressive writing in particular, among patients with HIV. One of the most striking was conducted by Keith Petrie, a psychologist at the University of Auckland School of Medicine in New Zealand. In his study, HIV patients randomly assigned to engage in expressive writing showed enhanced immune function, such as increased CD4 levels and lower viral load, up to six months after the intervention. A study by O'Cleirigh and colleagues examined the relationship between emotional expression and long-term survival rate of HIV/AIDS. They found evidence of some benefit of disclosure, with healthy long-term survivors showing more emotional disclosure than a comparison group of patients with HIV. Emotional disclosure was related to enhanced emotional and cognitive processing and better biological indicators of immune function (such as increased CD4 count, decreased viral load), but only in women.

Other studies have used variations on the typical writing study. For example, Traci Mann at the University of Minnesota conducted an ingenious study where she asked HIV-positive women to write about the future in a manner that was intended to increase positive expectations. As she hoped, writing about the future increased people's sense of optimism and, at the same time, reduced their reports of side effects from the medications they were taking. A 2013 study by Gail Ironson and colleagues supplemented traditional expressive writing with exercises to facilitate problem solving, enhance self-worth, and better understand their traumatic experiences in patients with HIV who also had elevated symptoms of PTSD. They found benefits of this enhanced expressive writing but only for women. Women asked to write reported feeling less depressed, exhibited lower anxiety and depression symptoms, and had lower HIV-related symptoms, compared to women not asked to write. Men in the expressive writing group showed little difference compared to men in the control group. Although two of these studies with HIV patients suggest that women are more receptive to the positive effects of expressive writing than men, it is not clear why this may be the case. It is particularly confounding as such a difference is often not observed (or is even reversed, with men benefiting more than women from expressive writing) in other studies not involving HIV. This result may reflect a complex interaction of social roles, desires, and expectations regarding disclosure, and attributes of the social context (e.g., access to supportive others), although careful study of this issue remains to be done.

CANCERS

Cancers reflect a broad group of related diseases characterized by excessive and nonproductive cell growth. Left unchecked, these growths (called tumors) can spread into the organs and/or tissues of the body, causing damage, dysfunction, or even death. Cancers are one of the leading causes of death in the world, and in the United States, despite considerable treatment advances being made in recent years.

Expressive writing has been used as a supplement to standard medical care in a number of studies with different groups of cancer patients. Given the overwhelming experience of a cancer diagnosis and subsequent treatments, many thought that expressive writing could help patients through these difficult times. The results from multiple studies are promising but not overwhelming. It's clear that writing is no panacea—it is not going to cure cancer and very likely will not change the course of the disease. With this said, there is some evidence that writing can help with adjustment to cancer. It can also help people's quality of life and how they are able to deal with the disease on a daily basis.

One relatively early study with cancer patients was conducted by Annette Stanton, a researcher at UCLA, and her colleagues. Stanton asked breast cancer patients to write about their deepest thoughts and feelings regarding their disease. She found that patients showed a significant reduction in cancer-related medical visits and reported fewer physical symptoms. As we have seen before, expressive writing led to many more investigations into whether expressive writing could help people adjust to cancer. Shortly after the initial study, a separate study found that writing about their experience with breast cancer led to an improvement in patients' overall quality of life. Yet, this was soon followed by another study finding that, for patients with metastatic breast cancer, expressive writing did not improve physical or psychological outcomes.

Although much of the expressive writing work in cancer has been done in patients with breast cancer, other cancers have been studied as well. Cindy Carmack, working with her research team at the MD Anderson Cancer Center, studied expressive writing in a controlled study of 40 patients with colorectal cancer. Those in the expressive writing condition experienced less distress and better quality of life in the months afterward. More recently, Stephen Lepore and his team at Temple University conducted a similar study. Contrary to their expectations, they found no evidence that writing helped patients adjust to cancer. Interestingly, Lepore's group tried out a new technique where patients both wrote and talked about issues surrounding their cancer. This "dual disclosure" method showed improvements in psychological well-being.

Complicating the picture a bit more, writing may be most helpful if the patient lacks other safe and supportive opportunities to disclose. Several studies have found that disclosure may help protect cancer patients from the negative effects of being too shy or otherwise unable to share their feelings with others. Perhaps expressive writing alone or coupled with some form of social sharing may help cancer patients' adjustment when they don't have other safe and supportive avenues for disclosure.

There have been several efforts to summarize all the available research information dealing with cancer and expressive writing using the meta-analysis method. Steve Lepore and colleagues conducted a meta-analysis in 2004, examining the effects of expressive writing used by patients with cancer. They concluded that expressive writing produced small, but reliable, improvements in well-being in three different types of cancer: renal, prostate, and breast. More recently, in 2014, Erin Merz's research team reviewed all the expressive writing and cancer studies and echoed this sentiment. They concluded that there is little or no evidence that expressive writing can lead to cancer-specific improvements (e.g., in medical or clinical outcomes) but that writing may help to improve sleep, reduce pain, and decrease use of medical services. They also concluded that patients who are socially constrained (lacking a safe and supportive outlet for interpersonal disclosure) may especially benefit from expressive writing.

CARDIOVASCULAR DISEASE AND DIABETES

Cardiovascular disease refers to a broad class of diseases that involve the heart or blood vessels. Cardiovascular disease is the leading cause of death in the United States and most of the world. This includes coronary heart disease and atherosclerosis, in which plaque builds up inside the coronary arteries. As these arteries supply blood to the heart, plaques can reduce or disrupt the supply of blood and oxygen to the heart, possibly resulting in chest pain or even a heart attack. Metabolic risk, sometimes called metabolic syndrome, refers to factors that raise people's risk for heart disease, type 2 diabetes, and stroke. Some of the most common risk factors include high blood pressure, high triglyceride levels, and obesity. Many metabolic risks are the results of our behaviors—notably eating habits, exercise/fitness, smoking, and alcohol consumption.

Somewhat surprisingly, there is relatively little work examining the effects of expressive writing on cardiovascular, metabolic, and related disorders. Some studies with predominantly healthy individuals find that writing can influence heart rate, blood pressure, and other emotional and physiological processes that, presumably, should be relevant for disease processes. The handful of good experiments with people suffering from chronic cardiovascular and/or metabolic disease includes the following.

Blood Pressure

One study conducted with people suffering from hypertension or high blood pressure was quite promising. Kimberly McGuire and her colleagues examined the effects of expressive writing in 38 community adults selected because they had persistently elevated blood pressure (mild to moderate hypertension). Those assigned to expressive writing showed greater decreases in blood pressure one month after writing than those in the control writing conditions. For those fans of blood pressure readings, the drops were modest—about 6 mm Hg systolic and 4 mm Hg diastolic.

Myocardial Infarction

Two ambitious studies have attempted to explore the use of expressive writing following a heart attack, also known as a myocardial infarction. Working with a group of colleagues, Rob Horne asked patients who had recently had their first heart attack to write about their thoughts and feelings about having a heart attack, or to write in a neutral way about daily activities. Five months after writing, those in the expressive writing condition had fewer medical appointments and were taking fewer prescription medications compared to the neutral writing group. The expressive writing group was more engaged in self-care activities and generally was doing better—they attended more cardiac rehabilitation sessions, reported fewer cardiac symptoms, and had lower blood pressure.

A similar study by David Hevey's team also tested expressive writing in patients who had experienced a heart attack. Hevey was particularly interested in health-related quality of life, an overall assessment of how the patient was doing with regard to recovering from the heart attack. Patients were again asked to write either about their thoughts and feelings related to their heart attack or about control topics. Expressive writing was related to higher health-related quality of life three months after writing. Interestingly, and consistent with findings from other domains, patients who both exhibited a tendency toward more negative moods and were more socially inhibited benefited more from expressive writing than those who were naturally more upbeat and optimistic.

Type 2 Diabetes

Evidence for whether or not expressive writing can help people with type 2 diabetes is very limited and still unclear. Only a handful of small and preliminary studies have been conducted. One such study, conducted in Italy, found that expressive writing led to better glycated hemoglobin, or HbA1c, levels, an objective measure of diabetic control, and substantially reduced psychological distress several months after writing (relative to those writing about neutral topics). In contrast, a very small recent study conducted in Great Britain found that expressive writing did not lead to any observable improvements for patients with type 2 diabetes in primary care and may have even resulted in some increases in reported depression symptoms.

MAJOR MENTAL DISORDERS

Within the medical and psychiatric communities, major mental disorders such as depression and schizophrenia are increasingly considered chronic health problems. It makes sense. They are indeed chronic in that, once people are diagnosed with a major mental disorder, the odds of the disease lingering for months or years or recurring multiple times over the life span are quite high. As with other chronic diseases, there is increasing evidence that depression and schizophrenia are associated with genetic predispositions and neurochemical imbalances. They also are exacerbated by life stressors.

Major Depressive Disorder

The most common mental health problem in many parts of the world is major depressive disorder, or unipolar depression. Large-scale international studies estimate that approximately 10 percent of the world's population will experience at least one clinical depression in life. The diagnosis of a major depression is associated with elevated risk of suicide and higher rates of a variety of physical illnesses.

Ten years ago, depression would have been part of a section on mental health. In recent years, there has been a growing awareness and discussion about the many biological underpinnings of depression, including insights from medicine, neuroscience, and other fields. There is a growing body of evidence that suggests extensive and close links between depression and the immune system, particularly inflammation. We have known for at least two decades that people who are deeply depressed are more prone to cancer progression and even heart attacks. The general thinking had been that depressed people were simply under more stress and stress accelerated other diseases. More recently, however, researchers have made some compelling discoveries suggesting that depression and inflammation, in particular the function of proinflammatory cytokines in the body, may exert bidirectional effects. That is, not only that depression may result in increases in inflammation throughout the body, but that inflammation in the body may directly increase depression. More generally, there is converging evidence that the nervous, endocrine, and immune systems are highly interconnected and may strongly—and bidirectionally—influence a wide range of mental disorders.

Given the relatively consistent links between expressive writing and improved outcomes associated with autoimmune disorders, one would assume there would be good evidence that writing could help combat depression. Surprisingly, there have been virtually no large studies to test this idea. One of the few studies was conducted by Katherine Krpan and her colleagues, who examined 40 people diagnosed with major depressive disorder. They found that depressed individuals assigned to write about their deepest thoughts and feelings surrounding an emotional event showed significant reductions in depression scores immediately after writing and over one month later, relative to those asked to write about emotionally neutral topics. We are unaware of any other high-quality studies that have carefully examined the use of expressive writing in people with major depression.

Looking beyond studies specifically with people diagnosed with a clinical disorder, some evidence for the benefit of expressive writing for feelings of depression and general distress has also been found in people who were not clinically depressed. For example, among university students expressive writing has been found to result in fewer depressive symptoms six months after writing. Expressive writing also has been shown to protect university students against upsetting intrusive or unwanted thoughts about stressful experiences and from ruminating about such experiences.

It is surprising that so few studies have been published on expressive writing and major depression (or, in fact, most other major mental disorders). In talking with clinical psychologists, several have expressed some anxiety about running such studies. For example, one theory of depression assumes that it is a disorder of self-awareness. People who are depressed use the word *I* far more than people who are not depressed. It is well known that depressed people are frequently looking inward, second-guessing their own thoughts and feelings, and ruminating about their shortcomings. Some clinicians consider expressive writing a form of therapy that encourages people to look inward. In their mind, the last thing that depressed people need is to look inward any more.

We trust the clinicians we have interviewed. As scientists, however, we hope that people interested in depression research begin experimenting with writing. Perhaps brief writing sessions might work, or one of the many variants of writing instructions that provide more guidance, focus on more positive aspects of experience in writing, and so forth. Given that the limited number of studies that have been conducted to date appear to have been at least somewhat successful, we hope we have more to report when the next edition of this book comes out.

Posttraumatic Stress Disorder

Remember the story of Joey, the Vietnam vet described in Chapter 3? It is generally believed that PTSD is the result of a major, often life-threatening, traumatic experience. PTSD is typically diagnosed when symptoms such as flashbacks, major sleep disruption, exaggerated fear and stress responses, memory problems, and feelings of depression and emotional numbness are severe and persist for months or longer following the event. Recent evidence suggests that there may be a genetic predisposition for the disorder that strongly increases the likelihood of developing PTSD following a traumatic experience.

Several small studies suggested that writing may help people with PTSD better manage their symptoms. Josh, along with several of his former students, found some benefit to expressive writing in a study of patients with PTSD. In that study, 25 patients with PTSD who had had traumatic war experiences or sexual assaults either completed an expressive writing intervention or wrote about emotionally neutral topics. Expressive writing improved people's mood, resulted in greater posttraumatic growth, and reduced physiological stress reactivity in response to their traumatic memories. A related study in the United

Kingdom by Mark Bernard and colleagues relied on a small clinical sample of 22 participants recovering from a first episode of psychosis with psychosis-related PTSD. Those instructed to write about the most stressful aspects of their illness had fewer avoidance symptoms, suggesting a lessening of the negative and traumatic impact of these experiences.

Much of the best work in the area of applying expressive writing to symptoms of PTSD and samples with actual PTSD diagnoses has been done by Denise Sloan, a researcher at Boston University, the National Center for PTSD, and the Veterans Administration. Denise is a clinical psychologist who has conducted many expressive writing studies with people struggling with PTSD symptoms. In an impressive study published in 2012, Denise and colleagues had survivors of serious motor vehicle accidents write about their experiences or write about superficial control topics. Compared to those in a control group, people in the expressive writing group had fewer PTSD symptoms in the months after writing. What made this study so noteworthy is that the actual rate of PTSD dropped in the emotional writing group but not in the control condition. In a later study, Sloan led a team that examined the effectiveness of expressive writing in a very small study of war veterans with PTSD. She found that PTSD symptom severity decreased in the months following the treatment. What's more, five of the seven veterans no longer met diagnostic PTSD criteria three months later.

It is important to note that not all studies have been this successful. Another study by Sloan's team found no significant treatment effects for people with PTSD; such differences may be due to the patients involved in the research (e.g., young students versus older veterans), the severity of PTSD symptoms, the cause of PTSD (motor vehicle accidents, war experiences, other), or many additional factors. Other researchers too have been unable to clearly document benefits of expressive writing to persons suffering with PTSD or PTSD symptoms. Although promising, we still need to better understand under what conditions expressive writing is a useful treatment for individuals with PTSD.

Bipolar Depression and Schizophrenia

Bipolar depression used to be called manic depression. Unlike unipolar depression, bipolar is strongly genetic and is often characterized by episodes of deep depression and, at other times, by highly agitated or manic states, often with periods of delusions. Historically, schizophrenia has been defined as a major thought disorder associated with blunted emotional reactions and delusional thinking styles. Interestingly, many people who have been diagnosed as bipolar by one expert have been diagnosed as schizophrenic by others. Over the last decade, advances in genetic research are beginning to suggest that there is substantial overlap in the genetic profiles of both bipolar disorder and schizophrenia. Making this story even more interesting, some of the same genes are linked to autoimmune function. Others are linked to creativity. For many people, then, these may be a single "diagnosis."

To date, we are unaware of any large-scale studies using expressive writing for either disorder. One reason is that in the midst of a full-blown depressive, manic, or schizophrenic episode, expressive writing may be ineffective. However, therapists and former patients have written to us reporting that expressive writing had been helpful when not in the midst of a psychotic episode. Okay, okay, we know this is just hearsay evidence. However, it may be well worth more carefully exploring in the future.

Final Thoughts on Expressive Writing for Chronic Disease

Let's say that you are dealing with a chronic disease and you think expressive writing might be good for you. What should you write about? Several of the studies described in this chapter had people write about their disease. Others had people write about the most traumatic experience of their lives. To be honest, the reason these two topics were used most of the time was that the scientists running the studies either wanted to make their writing study relevant to the group of people they were studying or wanted to be sure to stick to the original instructions used in the very first writing study published in 1986.

When Josh conducted his first big experiment with arthritis and asthma patients, he got a glimpse of the possible shortcomings of specific writing instructions when he read a comment by one of his participants, Nick. Nick was in his late 40s and was a plumber. He had been diagnosed a couple of years earlier with arthritis and was starting to experience fairly serious pain in his joints—especially his hands. Although in this study he was able to write about his arthritis, or other issues, he insightfully pointed to a larger issue:

> *I thought at first I would write about being sick. But that wasn't really the thing I wanted to write about. I've been sick a lot before. Even though I may not get better from this, that's not it. More it's that this makes me less a man. I worry that I won't be able to work. Use my hands. Take care of my family. Do things I want to. This sickness is going to take away who I am. And I can't tell anyone about it—they don't want to hear me bitch about it. Can't stress my wife out. Friends, not them too. They have their own problems to deal with, they don't need to hear about mine.*

Nick gets at the essential issues—expressive writing should work best when writing about issues that are most troubling. It may be something directly related to an illness, or it might be the impact of the illness—now or in the future—or important aspects of life, family, activities, whatever is important. And sometimes it might be something completely unrelated to the illness. He brings up an issue we have touched on already: writing is often most useful when someone doesn't have other opportunities to disclose.

If you are dealing with a chronic disease, write about whatever topics are bothering you most. A chronic disease arouses a mind-boggling number of issues that you may have never thought about before. The diagnosis and the symptoms could force you to think about your close relationships, financial concerns, disability, death, or new plans for the future. Remember that writing is for you and this might be an opportunity to explore these topics in an open and honest way that you haven't felt free to do before.

*   *   *

Many, many studies have now been conducted with patients dealing with chronic and sometimes life-threatening diseases. Dramatic stories about the benefits of writing regularly appear in the media (many overhyped, some quite balanced). Not all studies have been successful, others have. In some ways, this is entirely consistent with the haphazard way science works and how science news is disseminated. Cholesterol is bad. Not so bad. Bad again. Parts of it are bad. Things can get muddled pretty quickly. Some of the same issues occur with expressive writing. With each new study, we are learning more about limits to the writing technique as well as methods that boost its effectiveness. Rather than covering in detail the scores of studies dealing with dozens of diseases, we have focused on studies that are revealing about some of the broader issues of writing and long-term health.

Can expressive writing help people manage chronic conditions and improve health? Yes, probably, but there are many unanswered questions. What we do know is that there is great promise. Several very high-quality studies have shown that expressive writing, added to standard medical treatment/care, can improve serious medical illnesses including asthma, arthritis, HIV/AIDS, and PTSD. Writing can help people dealing with chronic medical conditions, either at diagnosis or in the ongoing management of a chronic or progressive illness, including cancers and possibly cardiovascular disease. Expressive writing may be useful when combined with psychotherapy, and helpful for people who don't have other supportive, safe, or helpful avenues of disclosure—perhaps due to the stigma of a disease (such as HIV), social constraints, or other reasons.

Writing won't cure cancer (or any other disease), and it may not help as much once a disease has progressed sufficiently so that biological systems are seriously compromised (that is, once a person has gotten too sick). For many other patients, however, writing may help enhance emotional, psychological, behavioral, and biological processes that, in turn, may contribute to improvements in health and well-being.

CHAPTER 5

Writing to Clear the Mind

EXPRESSIVE WRITING IN LEARNING AND EDUCATION

It's time for a break. Think of the topics that have been covered so far: massive, horrible personal traumas, death, loss, life-threatening illnesses, and the pain of splinters, depression, war. There is much more to expressive writing than overcoming the grim realities of life.

Expressive writing is usually enjoyable and meaningful. Across hundreds of studies, people report that they actually like to explore their thoughts and feelings. *And* they find that it can help them in all types of situations.

So let's lighten up. What are your thoughts about the Russian Revolution? How about the British East India Tea Company? Or country and western songs?

We don't need to talk to others to tell our untold stories. Whether we talk into an audio recorder, scribble on a magic pad, or type on our iPad, translating thoughts into language can be psychologically and physically beneficial. When people write about important events, they begin to organize and understand them. Writing about the thoughts and feelings connected with unexpected experiences forces us to bring together their many facets. Once we can distill complex experiences into more understandable packages, we can begin to move beyond them.

Writing, then, organizes upheavals. What about other complex experiences that are not traumatic? For example, if you were learning about all the factors that led to the Russian Revolution in 1917, would it help you to write about your feelings concerning what you were learning? Or, if you were in the process of beginning a new job, would it be beneficial to write about your experiences at the end of each day? Coming to terms with the Russian Revolution or a new job can be highly complicated tasks. If writing about a trauma helps to organize the experience, writing should work in the same way when we deal with any new tasks.

Writing as a Tool for Education

Consider the nature of education. The primary mission of high schools and colleges is to get students to understand and integrate ideas from a variety of disciplines. The goal of the educational system is largely to prepare students for the real world by training them to think more broadly. As teachers, we secretly hope that each of our eager students will assimilate what we tell them and, when we meet them later in life, they will thank us profusely for changing their worldviews. Why does this so rarely happen? The answer may lie, in part, in the distinction between confronting versus being confronted by events. Teachers often lecture, or psychologically confront, a large group of students with a bewildering number of facts, theories, and stories. The traditional role of the students is to be passive recipients of information. We confront them with information; they are confronted by it. In a twisted sort of way, a lecture is like a trauma for the audience. People are passively confronted by a bewildering amount of information over which they have very little control.

If we want students to assimilate the information we give them, we must change our educational strategies. Students should be actively encouraged to write or talk about our facts and theories. Even more powerful would be to have them write about relevant educational material within the context of their own personal experiences. Further, if exams are intended to stimulate learning rather than solely evaluate students' performance, multiple-choice exams should be outlawed. Essay exams, which actively promote the integration of information, should be encouraged.

AN IN-CLASS WRITING SYSTEM

In response to our investigations along these lines, Jamie developed a simple in-class writing strategy that demanded that students confront the reading and lecture material to which they had been exposed. One of the classes that he was teaching at the time was a team-taught course entitled "Social and Political Institutions from 1854 to the Present." This required class attempted to explain selected social, economic, and political institutions that had shaped the 20th century and created many of the current problems in the world. Although a potentially fascinating class, it had traditionally been disliked by students because of the overwhelming reading load and the seemingly unrelated lectures given in a rotating manner by one of five instructors from different disciplines.

In addition to two general lectures each week, students attended one weekly discussion section of about 30 people. In the section, the instructor attempted to generate an exciting intellectual debate about the topics of the week. The word *attempted* is apropos because most discussion sections didn't work very well, if at all. The students had been so inundated with reading and lecture material they couldn't sort the relevant from the irrelevant. It was in the discussion sections that the in-class writing system was introduced.

At the beginning of each discussion class, students were provided with a very brief overview of the main ideas of the readings and lectures. They were then asked to write continuously for 10 minutes about their deepest thoughts and feelings about the topic. Although students turned their writing assignments in to the instructor, they were never graded on what they wrote—no matter how crazy or offensive it was.

The transformation in the students was startling. Before writing, it was impossible to get a discussion going, unless it had nothing to do with the topic. After writing, however, almost all of the students contributed interesting and insightful ideas about formerly obscure topics—such as how the British East India Tea Company promoted the growth of imperialism in India. Their writing had forced them to assimilate ideas from a variety of sources as well as from their own experiences. All of a sudden, topics such as the British East India Tea Company or the plight of the Mosquito Indians in Guatemala became relevant to their own lives. Once the writing assignments had started, absentee rates dropped and performance on exams (essay, of course) improved dramatically. The irony is inescapable. The in-class writing assignment took about 10 minutes, or 20 percent, of each class period. The students were confronted with less information but learned much more (and more effectively) than students in regular classes.

The use of in-class writing to boost learning has become increasingly popular in recent years. A team of researchers led by Robert Bangert-Drowns at the University of Albany analyzed data from 48 school-based writing-to-learn programs. They found that small but reliable improvements in students' grades and other academic achievement measures. These benefits were more pronounced when the writing tasks pushed students to think broadly about their writing topics.

Particularly exciting is that there has been a concerted effort to see if writing skills training can help students with learning disabilities. Typically these students do not display strong writing skills, yet studies show that they function well conceptually. A meta-analysis by Gersten and Baker showed that teaching expressive writing to students with learning disabilities resulted in improved writing skills, self-efficacy, and creative thinking. Other projects have found that writing training not only improved writing skills but that performance in later courses continued to improve compared to that of students who had not had the writing training.

Writing to Improve Learning and Health Outcomes

More traditional expressive writing exercises have been used in educational contexts as well. A series of fascinating studies was conducted by Kitty Klein and Adriel Boals using expressive writing to track changes in working memory. Working memory refers to the ability of people to hold several ideas in memory at the same time. Students assigned to the expressive writing condition showed improvements in short-term working memory, suggesting an enhanced capacity to manage information, data, memory, and so forth. Working with a different group of students, Klein and Boals asked them to write about either positive topics or a challenging negative experience. Only those who wrote about challenging negative events showed improvements in working memory. Writing helped the students make sense of their experiences, reducing the need to think or ruminate about them and "freeing up" mental resources that allowed them to flourish in their college experience.

That writing about negative experiences may be more powerful than writing about positive ones is a contentious issue in the expressive writing world. There are now several experiments that suggest that writing about both positive and negative experiences can lead to better learning and health. For example, asking people to explore important issues in life and focusing on the potential benefits of these experiences can be helpful.

One factor may broker the debate about the relative merit of writing about negative or positive experiences: the amount of cognitive work or thinking the person must do about the topic. Putting complex ideas together requires effort. There is no doubt that making sense of a traumatic experience can tax our resources. Many positive experiences are no different. They can be overwhelming and can disrupt our entire lives. We typically don't think about "putting our lives back together" after a positive experience—but we actually *do* have to put our lives into some kind of new order afterward. Think of the biggest positive experiences in your life: new love, new job, new baby, a new house. They are generally great but disruptive events.

The importance of seriously thinking about life transitions in expressive writing was demonstrated in a study with stressed medical students. The authors asked the students to write about their thoughts and feelings about their lives. Those who showed more deep-level thinking along with constructive problem solving were less depressed later and had fewer health care visits. Those medical students who merely expressed their emotions and described their anxiety had more health care visits.

These findings square with a recent project exploring writing styles of over 25,000 students' college admissions essays and their later performance in college. Using computerized text analysis methods, Jamie and a group of his colleagues found that college admissions essays that revealed more formal and logical thinking predicted higher student grade-point averages over the entire time the students were in college. Logical thinking, rather than just telling stories, was the key to academic success.

ON THE TRAINING OF WRITING, READING, AND THINKING SKILLS

The role of writing in education was a hotly debated topic for most of the 20th century. Much of the controversy grew from the writings of Lev Vygotsky, a Soviet psychologist who died at the age of 38 in 1934. Vygotsky proposed new ways to understand language and thought in ways that continue to challenge traditional views of education.

Children, he argued, used language to sort out their thoughts and to solve real-world problems. In his view, young children naturally progressed through a series of phases that allowed them to communicate with others and, eventually, themselves. This progression began with noises and gestures, then spoken language, play, symbolic play in the form of drawing, and finally written language. Writing, then, meant going from drawing pictures to drawing words.

In a startling experiment with three- and four-year-olds, one of Vygotsky's colleagues, Alexander R. Luria, demonstrated that children understood the nature of writing even though they couldn't read. For example, Luria told the children to memorize a series of phrases. Once the children realized that there were too many phrases to remember, Luria handed them a pencil and paper and told them to write down what he was saying. Even though none of the children could write, they seemed to mimic writing behaviors that they had seen in adults. Most of the young children, then, would make little scribbles each time Luria called out a phrase. Later, when Luria asked each of the children to recall the words and phrases, many would look at the marks and squiggles and, according to Vygotsky (1978, p. 114), "repeatedly indicate, without error, which marks denote which phrase. . . . We are . . . seeing the first precursor of future writing."

The work of Vygotsky and Luria suggested that speaking and writing skills are fundamental to humans and partially dictate how we perceive the world. Vygotsky was adamant that the way children were taught to read and write, in both Russia and the West, should be changed. Writing, which he viewed as a symbolic form of drawing, was as basic as speaking. Because it was a natural development, children should be given the opportunity to learn to read and write as early as age three. But the method of learning should not be based on the imposed (confronted-by) rote teaching styles that most of us grew up with. Rather, reading and writing skills should be seen as desirable forms of communication by the children. For example, children should be shown that by writing, they can communicate their thoughts in letters or diaries. In short, Vygotsky argued that young children should confront writing skills rather than be confronted by them.

Much of Vygotsky's work has profoundly affected educators. For example, a range of educational projects emerged encouraging children to write in a stream-of-consciousness manner as early as the first grade. These writing techniques, variously called freewriting or process writing, often produced impressive gains in students' writing and reading abilities. Donald Graves, of the University of New Hampshire, spent many years developing a process writing program for young elementary school children. He has found that those who are expected to write freely about their personal experiences learn to read more quickly and to perform better on a variety of verbal tests.

A number of secondary and college educators, too, have been successfully exploring the benefits of freewriting. Peter Elbow, at the University of Massachusetts at Amherst, has been at the forefront of this movement in proposing how college students and adults can overcome writer's block and their general fears concerning writing. He finds that having people write continuously for 10 minutes a day serves as a mental conditioning technique. Indeed, for people who often have trouble writing—whether a paper for class or a report for the office—he finds that the 10-minute freewriting exercise can "jump-start" the brain. (Recall we asked you to try this exercise earlier in the book!)

Writing as a Boost to Learning and Creativity

As long as we are on the topic of writing and education, it makes sense to comment briefly on the art of taking notes. Note taking, whether in the classroom, in a business meeting, or when talking with a client, serves a similar function to writing in general. We usually take notes to help us remember the main points of a lecture or meeting.

Interestingly, notes can reflect either a *being-confronted-by* or a *confronting* strategy. When people are in a being-confronted-by mode, their notes usually focus on detail, including numerous direct quotes. Notes taken in this mode are almost transcriptions wherein the note-taker is not actively thinking during the lecture or talk. Notes taken with a confronting strategy, on the other hand, are much broader and integrative. The note-taker, who is actively thinking about the topic, will often write down a brief summary of what the speaker is discussing along with his or her own views on the matter.

Research on note-taking strategies by Gillis Einstein and his colleagues at Furman University indicates that students who perform the best on exams tend to adopt confronting methods of taking notes. Those who perform poorly typically focus on details, congruent with a being-confronted-by strategy. Other research finds that students who take "summarized" notes versus verbatim notes comprehend material better. Summarized notes foster the process of transforming the information into something meaningful, which helps students integrate new information with previously known information.

It is not coincidental that the being-confronted-by approach is a form of low-level thinking that often occurs when people are in uncontrollable or unpredictable situations. Individuals who adopt a low-level thinking style, not unlike those using a being-confronted-by mode of note taking, tend to focus on details, adopt a narrow time perspective, and are unable to self-reflect.

Like drawing, writing is a natural human activity. One of its values is in helping us integrate and organize our complicated lives. Writing accomplishes this less-than-modest goal in a variety of ways:

- *Writing clears the mind.* Before beginning a complex task, it can be beneficial to write out your thoughts and feelings. Indeed, many professional hypnotists often use this technique to accelerate the hypnotic procedure. Basically, they ask their clients to jot down their current thoughts and feelings. When their clients finish writing, the hypnotists tell them to tear up the paper and throw it away. This serves as a symbolic form of clearing the mind.

- *Writing resolves troublesome experiences that stand in the way of important tasks.* Following major upheavals, people tend to obsess about them. In thinking about the traumas, and even in trying not to think about them, individuals use a great deal of their thinking capacity. They become forgetful and cannot sustain their attention on large new tasks. Writing about traumas helps to organize the traumas, thereby freeing the mind to deal with other tasks.

- *Writing helps in acquiring and remembering new information.* As the note-taking research indicates, writing thoughtful notes or, in the case of young children, squiggles, helps people take in and recall new ideas. Writing can help provide a framework by which to understand the new and unique perspectives of others. Indeed, writing about them makes the ideas more vivid and memorable.

- *Writing fosters problem solving.* Because writing promotes the integration of information, it can help us solve complex problems. If people write freely about a complicated problem they are dealing with, they can more readily find a solution. There are several reasons for this. One is that writing forces people to sustain their attention on a given topic for a longer period than they normally would do if they were just thinking about it. Because writing is slower than thinking, each idea must be thought about in greater detail. Writing is also more "linear" than thinking in that writing forces an entire idea to be transcribed before another is entertained.

• *Freewriting promotes forced writing.* Most people are called on to write something on occasion—whether a legal brief, a medical opinion, or a letter of complaint to the city dog catcher. Formal writing can be a serious drag. Every sentence can sound stilted, every word inappropriate. Freely writing your thoughts and feelings before beginning any formal writing can loosen your writing skills. Even using freewriting as the basis of a rough draft can be helpful.

There is no need to belabor the point further. Writing can be an invaluable skill in learning about and coping with the world. Under the right circumstances, writing promotes mental and physical health. Although it won't work for everyone all the time, the judicious use of writing can improve the quality of life for many of us.

Writing for Problem Solving

As noted in the text, writing can help with effective problem solving. For this exercise, write down a problem you are facing. Write freely, as with other exercises, without regard to spelling or grammar, for about 10 minutes. Review your writing and identify the key impediments or barriers—now write about these, again for about 10 minutes. Finally, reread both sets of writing—and write a final time, again for 10 minutes, synthesizing your thoughts and insights about the problem, barriers to overcoming it, and identify potential solutions or ways to solve the problem. Sometimes, this exercise may give rise to immediate insights (or even a solution), but often it facilitates a process that yields a solution in time.

Diaries, Journals, and Social Media

Given that writing has so many apparent benefits, you would think that people who keep diaries would be wonderfully happy, healthy, and creative. Sadly, the world is not so simple and straightforward. There is a good reason for this. The ways people keep and use diaries is amazingly diverse.

In our surveys of thousands of college students, for example, over 50 percent never write in a diary or journal. Another 40 percent or so write in a diary once or twice a week. Only about 3 percent write daily or almost daily. Although women in our samples tend to use diaries more than men, the gender difference is surprisingly small. Of particular importance is that frequent diary writers are no healthier than people who rarely or never use diaries.

One reason it is hard to evaluate the health effects of diary writing is that we don't know what the diary writers' health would be if they didn't write in their diaries. Who knows? Maybe diary writers are staving off a plethora of dreaded diseases by writing. Similarly, there may be fundamental personality differences between people who do and don't keep a diary. Perhaps people who don't use diaries are more socially at ease and can talk about their deepest thoughts and feelings to others. Maybe they just don't need to rely on a diary. Finally, it is always difficult to sort out the motivations for people keeping diaries. Some may have been inspired by Samuel Pepys and the detailed confessional and descriptive diaries that he kept for 10 years of his life in the 17th century. Others may be required to maintain a diary because of religious doctrine. Many simply want a record of whom they have seen and what they have done in their lives.

A more intriguing issue, however, is what people decide to put in their diaries and journals. Mormons, for example, strongly encourage their members to maintain a diary of their lives. Indeed, the Mormons have assembled one of the most impressive genealogical libraries in the Western Hemisphere, which houses many of these journals. The journals are typically factual and not emotional. That is, most Mormons who keep diaries do not explore their most secret or personal thoughts, probably because they know that their diaries may be read for generations after their death.

Among the people we have interviewed who have kept intimate and emotional diaries, two distinctly different patterns have emerged in the ways they maintain their diaries. One group writes only during periods of stress or unhappiness. If life is plodding along in a fairly predictable way, people in this group simply have no interest in writing. The second group, which is less than half the size of the first, writes almost daily. That is, until traumas strike. During massive stressors, people in the second group typically stop writing. For example, one well-adjusted woman, who had written almost daily for years, abruptly stopped writing the day she learned of her daughter's unexpected death. She explained that she could talk about the death but could not yet write about it. In fact, she did not begin exploring her thoughts and feelings on paper until a year and a half after the death.

Oddly, neither Josh nor Jamie has met a person who wrote about his or her deepest feelings who did not fall generally into one of these two writing patterns. We are certain that there are some exceptions. We just haven't met one yet. The apparent existence of these two writing patterns suggests the different functions writing can serve for people. For those who write only during or following a trauma, diaries may serve as a way to cope—perhaps as a substitute for talking with others about the traumas. Those in the second group, who stop writing during times of trauma, report that the emotions are too intense to deal with in journal form.

Finally, at least until recently, there existed a separate group—people who regularly write letters to others. Interestingly, letter writers typically do not classify themselves as diary or journal writers, but, in writing their letters, they very often explore their deepest thoughts and feelings on an almost daily basis. The major difference between diary and letter writing is the degree to which the writers feel free to disclose intimate parts of themselves, with letter writers usually sending the letters to a recipient. A novel twist on letter writing has emerged, with the advent of a hybrid category of letter disclosure facilitated by computer and technological advances—people writing to others whom they typically don't know, often anonymously.

Adding Computers to the Mix

Perhaps the most interesting and important development in the letter-writing tradition has been the advent of the computer and Internet. Starting with computerized/electronic bulletin boards, and progressing through chat rooms to Facebook and other social media outlets, people now have a near limitless opportunity and potential audience for their "letters." Individuals can write long letters or short notes proclaiming their views on politics, physics, or love. What makes online writing so novel is that people's letters can be anonymous. Online expressions, then, are a little like talking to someone on an airplane. Consequently, people often disclose some of their very deepest feelings.

Is writing in a blog format good for you? In a series of stunning articles by Azy Barak and his colleagues at Haifa University in Israel, the answer appears to be yes. In one of their most persuasive studies, Barak recruited 161 adolescents between the ages of 14 and 17 who were suffering from social or emotional difficulties at school or elsewhere. He then randomly assigned students to write about their difficulties either on a public blog or just on their computer so that no one else could see their writing. Others either didn't write or just wrote in a stream-of-consciousness way. The students were asked to write at least twice a week for 10 weeks. The results were quite strong: students who wrote in public blogs showed the most improvements in social behaviors and drops in social anxiety.

It turns out that these benefits are not limited to blogs. Barak also finds that students who use instant messaging (IM) to describe their thoughts and feelings evidence drops in anxiety and better adjustment. Indeed, his lab has summarized over 60 studies of people using online psychotherapy (which relies on e-mail or other electronic communication). Overall, online therapy appears to be as beneficial as traditional face-to-face therapy.

With this said, all is not rosy on the Internet—although hundreds of millions of people use Facebook each day, presumably in part sharing their thoughts and feelings with others, it may not be helpful. In a fascinating study from 2013, Ethan Kross at the University of Michigan and an international team of collaborators studied the effects of Facebook use in young adults—the heaviest users. In brief, they found that the more people used Facebook over two weeks, the more their life satisfaction declined. In fact, even individual Facebook sessions were associated with feeling worse several hours later! This is not to say that using Facebook will necessarily make you miserable, but that not all "social" interactions online are helpful.

The Downside of Writing

In our excitement about our research findings we may seem to have portrayed writing as a cure for everything. An uncritical reading of this book would give the impression that writing about your deepest thoughts and feelings will inevitably make you physically healthier, mentally alert, smarter, and the epitome of psychological health. Yes, writing can be quite healthy. But an overreliance on writing can pose some problems—at least in some situations. In evaluating your own writing, be sure to ask yourself the following questions.

ARE YOU USING WRITING AS A SUBSTITUTE FOR ACTION?

Writing may be particularly suited to and effective in dealing with issues that are uncontrollable. After a death or other trauma, writing helps us sort out complicated feelings and memories. In potentially controllable situations, however, writing may be counterproductive. That is, if we can do something to change an unpleasant situation, we are much better off changing it than merely writing about it.

In one of our writing experiments, for example, one woman wrote during each session about how much she disliked her roommate. Her roommate, according to her essays, was messy, borrowed her clothes without asking, and talked on the phone too much. Gleaning from what she wrote, her strategy in dealing with her roommate's behavior was to stay away from her own room as much as possible. One can't help wondering what would have happened if the two women had been able to sit down and discuss the nature of their problems with each other.

IS YOUR WRITING AN INTELLECTUAL RATHER THAN A SELF-REFLECTIVE EXERCISE?

A few years ago, a gentleman in his 40s contacted one of us because he was experiencing a tremendous amount of stress from his job and marriage. Both his physical and mental health were suffering even though he had been writing daily for several months—writing he was eager to share. He was a fluid writer with an impressive vocabulary and a keen eye for nuances in people's behaviors. In his writing, he drew heavily from Jung, Spinoza, Aristotle, Lao-Tzu, and other intellectual luminaries. Despite his insight into other people's behaviors and even his own mental processes, he never wrote about his own emotions or why he felt the way he did. He was so concerned with demonstrating his own brilliance that he forgot why he was writing in the first place.

It's grand to be smart. But intelligence and a classical education do not guarantee anyone emotional stability or personal insight. If you find that your writing often moves in a safe and nonpersonal direction wherein you are citing the work of Virginia Woolf to explain the ultimate failure of Napoleon, your writing may be quite interesting and even publishable. But don't expect intellectualization to improve your health.

ARE YOU USING WRITING AS A FORUM FOR UNCENSORED COMPLAINING?

Remember that a prime value of writing is that it forces us to ask how and why we feel the ways we do. Ideally, writing helps us organize, structure, order, and make meaning of these experiences. As a self-reflective exercise, it is beneficial to acknowledge our deepest emotions and thoughts. If your lover has left you for someone else, it would undoubtedly be helpful to explore why you feel so bereft, so lonely, or so angry. Merely complaining about your cruel ex-lover will not be particularly healing. Indeed, it may be harmful.

Many studies have demonstrated that blindly venting anger often makes us feel angrier. Hitting a pillow, pretending it is someone we would like to slug, usually increases our blood pressure and encourages us to think of alternative or additional acts of vengeance. Talking or writing about the source of our problems without self-reflection merely adds to our distress. If you find that your writing focuses more on another person than on yourself, stop and ask yourself some questions. Why are you writing this way? How do you feel about what you are writing? Why does the other person bother you as he or she does?

And this brings us to a related point: overdisclosing. Some people, with no provocation at all, immediately disclose extremely intimate events in their lives. Not only to us, but they confess the same detailed events to virtually all of their friends, coworkers, and even passersby. Together, Jamie and Josh have interviewed perhaps half a dozen who fit this category. All have suffered from major health problems, including uterine cancer, ulcers, and glandular imbalances. Indeed, they disclose their health problems with the same relish as their traumas. In all cases, their disclosure is automatic, dramatic, and usually shocking for the listener.

Although these overdisclosers appear to be confiding their deepest thoughts and feelings, a closer analysis suggests that they are divulging traumatic events in a repetitive fashion without self-reflecting. Again, they have rehearsed the events in their minds and in conversations thousands of times, but have not explored either their emotions or the meanings of the events to their lives. Overdisclosing, then, is much like a verbal form of obsessive thinking. People talk or write about various aspects of a trauma without integrating the pieces or making any progress in making sense of their experiences.

IS YOUR WRITING AN EXERCISE IN SELF-REFLECTION OR IN SELF-ABSORPTION?

Periodically, and following a major upheaval, it is valuable for people to stand back and reflect on who they are, why they behave in the ways they do, and how and why they respond emotionally. Self-reflection provides a form of feedback so that individuals can decide whether they need to adjust their life course. Whereas periodic self-reflection is healthy, it can be carried to an extreme.

Let's be honest. We could ponder the meaning of an infinite number of events in our lives. Why, for example, did I just take a sip of coffee? How do I feel about that? What does that say about my childhood? And my feelings of security? Once we begin analyzing our deepest thoughts and feelings about everything, our self-absorption takes over our lives. During periods of self-reflection, we are, by definition, looking at ourselves to the exclusion of others. If we live completely in this self-reflective state, we cannot be empathic, a good friend or listener to others, or a useful member of society. To the degree that writing helps us understand and reorient our lives, it is beneficial. When we self-reflect to the point of self-absorption, it becomes maladaptive.

Final Thoughts on Writing to Clear the Mind

There is nothing magical about *writing* in a self-disclosing manner. It works much the same way as talking to others but without many of the social ramifications. Therein are its strengths and weaknesses. You cannot be punished or humiliated by writing per se. But you also cannot get feedback from others. Other people's views and opinions usually ground us in reality. Without consulting others, we can blow many of our thoughts and emotions far out of proportion—others can help provide us a "reality check" that we often need.

Writing should not serve as a substitute for friends. Many times, you may not be able to talk with others about particularly upsetting experiences. In these cases, writing can be quite helpful. Friends, however, can offer emotional support, advice, and other forms of assistance in ways that writing just can't do. Just because you may not be able to talk to some of your friends about a specific topic, remember that they are available for general advice and friendship. If friends are unavailable, psychotherapists and other people in the helping profession will listen to your problems and help keep your sense of reality intact.

Throughout this book, we have made numerous comparisons between writing and therapy. Both approaches can yield measurable improvements in psychological and physical health. Both encourage self-reflection and the attainment of insight about thoughts and moods. Both promote the acknowledgment and understanding of emotions.

To the degree that writing and therapy are used with basically healthy and well-adjusted people, the two techniques may provide similar advantages. The similarities, however, often stop here. For people who are deeply distressed and who are unable to cope effectively, therapy is often the only realistic alternative. When extremely distraught, individuals are often unable to write or think at all clearly or objectively. Similarly, when individuals suffer from a significant health problem, writing (or therapy) may positively influence their bodies. In most cases, however, they will be much wiser to visit a physician first. Antibiotic medications, for example, work more quickly and far more efficiently in dealing with infections than writing sessions.

Writing, then, should be viewed as preventive maintenance. The value of writing or talking about our thoughts and feelings lies in reducing the work of inhibition and in organizing our complicated and messy mental and emotional lives. Writing helps to keep our psychological compass oriented. Writing can be an inexpensive, simple, albeit sometimes painful way to help maintain our health.

CHAPTER 6

"Get These Thoughts Out of My Head!"

GETTING PAST OBSESSIONS, INSOMNIA, AND BOUTS OF STUPIDITY

A distinguished-looking businessman, about 45 years old, sat down next to Jamie for a flight from Boston to Dallas. While the plane taxied to take off, the two chatted about the weather and the traffic in Boston versus Dallas. The businessman was on his way to Dallas to attend a sales meeting related to office furniture. On learning that Jamie was a psychologist, he laughed nervously and assured him that he was as "fit as a fiddle." Except for an occasional headache.

And some problems with insomnia. Oh, and sometimes, waves of tension or nervousness.

It was nothing, really. It had lasted only about six or seven months. About the time that he and his wife had started remodeling their house. And the carpenter always seemed to be around. And whenever he was on a sales trip—which was quite often—his wife frequently wasn't home when he called at night. Even after he spotted his wife and the carpenter embracing in the backyard, he decided not to say anything. He was certain that his wife was having an affair.

They hadn't been in the air 20 minutes and the businessman had disclosed more about his thoughts and fears than he had to anyone in years. He described his recurring intrusive thoughts and emotions concerning his wife, the carpenter, and himself. Forbidden thoughts of suicide, murder, failure, and humiliation had become more and more frequent. Commuting to and from work, lying in bed at night, even in meetings, vivid images flashed before him.

He explained how he had tried to stop these thoughts. His attempts to keep busy all of the time didn't work. He was exercising heavily and consuming more alcohol. However, the images and emotions kept returning. Although distressed, the man on the plane was quite sane. Due, in part, to his reluctance to discuss his marital problems with anyone, he had become a prisoner of his own thoughts.

Where do such unwanted thoughts come from? How can we escape from them?

Prisoners of Unwanted Thoughts

Most people suffer from intrusive and unwanted thoughts at some points in their lives. Surveys of adults and college students indicate that the majority of unwanted thoughts deal with sex, aggression, illness and death, failure, relationship problems, dirt and contamination, and food. A closer examination of unwanted or obsessive thoughts reveals that people become prisoners of their own thoughts at fairly predictable times in their lives. Most unwanted thoughts begin to surface soon after an emotional upheaval or when they are reminded of an upheaval that may have occurred earlier in their lives.

The biggest danger of unwanted thoughts is that they can become larger and more threatening the more we dwell on them. A common unwanted thought among new parents, for example, concerns images of hurting their babies. Many new parents think to themselves, "What would other people say if they knew I had these murderous thoughts?" The thoughts then expand from harming the baby to overarching negative beliefs about themselves—"I am a horrible person." Their original thoughts, which were quite normal, soon go out of control.

People will often engage in a variety of behaviors to try to block the thoughts from their minds. Case studies have found that people can develop a fear of knives based on their thoughts of harming the baby and demand that all sharp instruments be removed from the house. Others, in coping with these unwanted thoughts, insist that another person always be present whenever the baby is around. Some simply become compulsively organized or throw themselves into a project of some kind—which helps to block the thoughts altogether.

A key symptom of anxiety and depression is rumination. Rumination involves reliving experiences and emotions that sufferers are trying to avoid. The more work people put into suppressing these thoughts, the more they return to consciousness. Does rumination cause depression or vice versa? The current thinking is that they go hand in hand and either can exacerbate the other.

Do You Ruminate Too Much?

This exercise will give you a rough estimate of how intensely or frequently you tend to ruminate. For each statement below, select the answer that best fits you using this scale. Answer each question as to how you typically are, not how you would like things to be.

0	1	2	3
Rarely true	Sometimes true	Often true	Very often true

When I'm sad, I continue to think about how bad I feel.

When something upsets me, I replay it in my mind for a long time.

I worry about bad things that could happen in the future.

I relive my embarrassing or awkward moments again and again in my mind.

I dwell on my problems for long periods of time.

Total up the numbers associated with your five selected answers. If you scored between 7 and 10, you likely have a tendency to engage in nonproductive rumination. If you scored above 10, your rumination may be common and/or intense enough to cause you distress.

At various times in our lives, all of us have had sexual, murderous, and even suicidal thoughts. Usually, these thoughts are not a problem in and of themselves. However, if the idea of having a particular thought is so repugnant, so threatening, so unacceptable that we immediately try to censor the thought, we may find that it returns to haunt us.

Much of the problem, then, is not our having unique or perverse

thoughts. Rather, one danger is trying to suppress the thoughts themselves. The more we try to suppress thoughts, the more likely it is that
they will resurface in our minds. The "white bear dilemma" is a perfect example.

Try not to think about a white bear.

No, seriously. Try not to think of one for the next minute or so. If
you really try this little thought experiment, you will probably fail. At
one time or another, some aspect of a white bear will appear in your
mind. This example comes from a fascinating line of studies originally
conducted by the legendary Harvard professor Dan Wegner. Across
several experiments, Wegner found that people have great difficulty
burying their unwanted mental images and thoughts.

Given the difficulty of suppressing thoughts of white bears, imagine the effort involved in trying to control images of unacceptable sexual perversions, the death of your child, or the murder of your spouse.
Wegner argued that the problem of suppressing psychologically
threatening thoughts is multiplied when we are depressed. When we
are happy, it is relatively easy to put a negative thought out of our
minds. If we are depressed or under stress, negative thoughts build on
themselves. Each attempt to suppress them tends to backfire, thereby
making the person even more depressed. Recent work has continued
to explore this paradox and has come up with the very impressive—
yet ominous—sounding label of "perseverative cognition" to explain
this process.

Is there any way out of the cycle? Once we are suffering from
recurring unwanted thoughts, is there some psychological trick that
allows us to break away? Well, yes and no. Some techniques we now
know do not work. Others are effective some of the time. Viktor
Frankl was one of the first people to note that a good way to overcome
unwanted thoughts was to stop trying to inhibit them. He encouraged patients to actively try to think about their unwanted thoughts.
His technique, typically referred to as paradoxical intention, has been
found to be effective in the treatment of obsessions.

Later in his career, Wegner proposed the *ironic process theory*,
which argued that thought suppression was both hard work and
almost impossible to accomplish because of the way the mind works.
Many people use distractions to try to suppress thoughts. For example,
they might take a shower or clean windows to escape from unwanted
thoughts. When these tasks don't sustain attention, however, the

thoughts wander back to the suppressed thought. Ultimately, these distractions remind people of the suppressed thought.

To complicate all of this, we naturally check ourselves to see how we are doing on any task. If we are trying not to think of a white bear, our mind can't help but periodically ask itself, "How am I doing in not thinking of the white bear?" And you can see the problem. The mind has just reminded itself of the white bear. Ironic, isn't it? No wonder Wegner called this his *ironic process model.* You can immediately see how problematic this can be when people are trying to suppress thoughts related to major traumas. Indeed, this has been an explanation of the thought cycles that people coping with PTSD struggle with.

The moral of this research may indeed be something you don't want to hear. If you are suffering from forbidden or unacceptable thoughts, you must allow yourself to think about them. Stop stopping. Making an unacceptable thought acceptable is the first step to moving toward more healthy thinking.

Building Healthier Thinking: Using Your Brain to Its Full Potential

Are there really such things as healthy versus unhealthy ways to think? Such a question presupposes that we know how to measure and define thinking styles in the first place. Nevertheless, if we could measure thinking styles, we could see if they helped to protect people against the adverse effects of stress in general or specific traumas they may have experienced.

The definition and measurement of thinking styles has dogged psychologists for generations. One of the earliest explanations evolved from research on the frontal cortex—the brain area known to be related to planning and complex thinking. The idea was that people who were more responsible, conscientious, and thoughtful were ultimately more psychologically healthy and resilient. To measure these qualities, neuropsychologists proposed a variety of tests to tap the workings of the frontal cortex—originally called executive function tests and more recently referred to as working memory tests. There are multiple versions of working memory tests. The basic idea is to see how much information you can juggle in your memory across a number of simple tasks.

Test Your Working Memory

There are many kinds of working memory tests. Below is a simple one that you can try on your own.

First, take 30 seconds or so and examine the follow sequence of numbers, trying to remember them:

$$1 \quad 3 \quad 2 \quad 3 \quad 7 \quad 4 \quad 8 \quad 2 \quad 5 \quad 9 \quad 6$$

Next, get ready to close the book—you are going to picture your three favorite animals, one after the other, for 5 seconds each, and then try to recall the original list of numbers—in order. You can write the numbers down on a scrap of paper. If you want a challenge, try to recall them in reverse order (the last number first, and so forth). Go ahead and try it, then come back to the book when you are done.

All done? Compare what you were able to recall with the numbers above. The more numbers you can recall, the better your working memory. In particular, if you can recall the numbers in order, you have a good working memory. Most people can recall about half of the numbers in order, with very few being able to recall them all.

What is interesting about tests such as these is that people do more poorly when they are under a great deal of stress than when they are stress free. Similarly, people who are depressed or ruminating about upsetting experiences perform more poorly on working memory tests.

We have already mentioned in passing two wonderful studies conducted in 2001 by Kitty Klein and Adriel Boals at North Carolina State University on expressive writing and working memory, but the details deserve more attention. They recruited around 140 first-year college students and, at the beginning of the semester, gave them weekly working memory tests. In addition, half the students were asked to write about their deepest thoughts and feelings about coming to college for four consecutive days, whereas the remainder of students wrote about superficial topics. What they discovered was that those who wrote about coming to college showed improvements in working memory.

But wait. It gets more interesting. Those who were in the expressive writing condition and whose working memory increased ended up making higher college grades during their first year of college. This is not an isolated finding. There have now been several studies finding that expressive writing improves students' grades. There have even been studies demonstrating that expressive writing in the days before major academic testing exams—such as the SAT or GRE—can improve people's performance on these tests.

One of the appeals of the working memory research is that it fits nicely into our commonsense models of how the brain works. When we are under stress, our minds are cluttered with thoughts and feelings that get in the way of our lives. We don't think as well. We are more forgetful. We do not pay as close attention to our environments. We become clumsier and more error prone. Ruminating and beating ourselves up just make matters worse.

Expressive writing or other measures to get ourselves to "stop stopping" are effective in cleaning out the clutter and allowing us to get on with life.

Getting Stupid to Avoid Stress

A friend who taught in the English department dropped by Jamie's office. He explained in a flat voice that his wife of 22 years had recently moved out "to try something new." Although he claimed not to be too distressed, consider what he was doing to avoid thinking about his wife. Usually a little sloppy, Peter confessed that he was vacuuming his entire house two or three times a day. He had stopped writing a book that was important to him. Rather than writing, he had devoted the last several days to checking his bank statements to be sure the bank hadn't made an error.

Most shocking was the change in his general thinking style. One reason Peter was a friend is that we enjoyed talking about books and articles. Peter, being a voracious reader and broad thinker, has the uncanny ability to tie together ideas from literature, anthropology, and related fields. As he talked, Peter maneuvered the topic of conversation away from his wife to a highly acclaimed book he had recently read. His analysis of the book caused Jamie's jaw to drop. In Peter's view, the book had some major problems: several instances of dangling participles, a few questionable spellings, and some incomplete sentences. But what about the general tone, the book's reflections on a generation influenced by drugs, television, and anomie? Peter wasn't interested in these issues. Rather, the dangling participle problem was far more urgent.

Escaping Uncontrollable Stress

When dealing with upsetting experiences, our working memory is reduced and, at the same time, our focus of attention is narrowed. We tend to think more narrowly and rigidly. By narrowing his focus to specks of dust on rugs, bank statements, and sentences rather than books, Peter was able to tune out some of the pain that he was experiencing. The work of trying to block unpleasant thoughts and emotions had taken its toll, however. The quality of his work suffered, as did his relationships with other people. Peter's mindlessness had alleviated the pain at the cost of his becoming temporarily stupid.

Peter's behavior is typical of many people facing massive uncontrollable stressors. In one study, for example, researchers examined the behaviors of Israeli women whose husbands were listed as missing in action during the 1973 Arab–Israeli war. A common response among the women was a compulsive preoccupation with trivial problems such as paying bills, choosing a carpet, and the like. By moving to extremely low levels of thought the women were actively avoiding thinking about a potentially devastating event.

Historically, several investigators have studied how thinking patterns change when people are under stress. Freud, for example, discussed a number of defense mechanisms that individuals employ to protect themselves from overwhelming feelings of anxiety. Many defense mechanisms, such as denial, suppression, and obsessions, are akin to low-level thinking strategies.

Across several studies, we know that when people are mindless, they perform more poorly on tests of creativity and complex thinking. Mindless people are also far more likely to be persuaded by con artists, television advertisements, and political speeches. In a very real sense, mindlessness makes us stupid.

Mindlessness is a thinking style that can protect us from feeling and thinking. If our lives are miserable, any escape can sometimes be welcome. Most of the examples suggest that low-level thinking reflects an automatic way of dealing with upsetting experiences. Usually, people move to lower thinking levels without any conscious awareness. As in the case of Peter, the English professor, as soon as he was separated from his wife, he automatically moved to a low level. Indeed, he wasn't even aware of his mindless behavior.

Low-level thinking in the service of avoiding stress or unwanted thoughts requires work. Sun Yee, whose husband of 40 years died suddenly, allowed us to read her diary several years later. In an entry written 10 days after his death, Sun Yee points to the psychological struggle of dealing with the pain:

I went back to work today. . . . It was good therapy—I cleaned the desk and organized the papers like a madwoman, but when I got home I fell apart. There's so much to tell and share, and no one to share it with. [Two days later] . . . The hardest times at the office are when I do automatic work, when I can think while I'm doing. Given a task that needs thinking through, I get involved and absorbed. Given a pack of cards to alphabetize, I cry. I remember how he used to call me during the day, cheery and loving and full of plans.

Whereas Sun Yee was tremendously insightful about her behavior and could structure her day to minimize her grief, many people turn to specific hobbies or habits that force a sustained lower thinking level.

What kind of hobbies or habits might do this? Both Josh and Jamie have long been interested in exercising. In recent years, people around the world have turned to jogging, racquet sports, weight lifting, and exercise groups to maintain their health and, perhaps, avoid dying. We suspect that this exercise craze also provides an efficient way to get stupid (i.e., move to a lower level of thinking).

We both speak from experience. During the most stressful periods of our lives, Josh has become a crazed tennis player, and Jamie has derived great enjoyment from long-distance jogging. Problems at work or at home disappear as soon as we begin sweating. Indeed, in the midst of a game or running, we are unable to concentrate for more than a few seconds on anything. Even if we wanted to, we could not contemplate the meaning of life, our deepest thoughts and feelings about love and death, or even how to rearrange our desks. While exercising, we might be in physical pain, but we are temporarily less distressed and more stupid.

As much fun as it is to taunt exercise fanatics, running and other forms of exercise—at least when done in moderation—provide a healthy form of escape from the stressors of daily life. Indeed, exercise is a far healthier way to delve into mindlessness than most of the alternatives. Alcohol and many psychoactive drugs are abused because they are quick and efficient in transporting the user to a lower level of thinking. Under the influence of alcohol, most people are incapable of being too self-reflective or aware of their own emotions, or grappling with complex psychological problems.

Finally, there are a host of psychological addictions that are, in effect, low-level thinking inducers. People completely immersed in their jobs (workaholics), in their eating and dieting patterns (food-aholics), sexual conquests (sexaholics), or even relationships with others often use their jobs, eating, sex, or whatever to avoid thinking about relevant psychological issues in their lives.

From Mindlessness to Mindfulness

Scientists have been attempting to identify how thinking patterns may influence our capacity to engage in effective problem solving for many years. One line of this work began in the mid-1970s, when Harvard psychologist Ellen Langer began a compelling project that sought to understand when people became "mindless" versus "mindful" in their everyday thinking. When people are mindless, they are rigid in their thinking and cannot appreciate novel approaches to problems. When mindful, people are active problem solvers, looking at the world from a variety of perspectives. According to Langer, all of us can be mindful at one time and mindless at others. Being mindless has some major drawbacks.

Soon after Langer published her first work on mindfulness, Jon Kabat-Zinn at the University of Massachusetts built a program to treat people with chronic illness using a different approach to mindfulness. Drawing on a Buddhist perspective, Kabat-Zinn suggested that mindfulness existed when a person was highly alert and attentive to a single experience. Whether the mindful person pays attention to his or her breathing or to the smell of a rose, the mind is still, focused, and centered.

In large part because of Kabat-Zinn's influence, there has been an explosion of interest in mindfulness in both the popular and scientific literatures. An impressive number of studies point to the health benefits of being mindful. Mindfulness, whether it is someone's general disposition or temporary state of being, is associated with more positive mental health and well-being. On the surface, Kabat-Zinn's meditative type of mindfulness sounds different from someone with a great deal of working memory who is engaged in everyday life. In fact, they are very similar in some ways. All types of mindfulness are best achieved when people do not have to actively monitor their thoughts or actions or relive horrible life experiences over and over.

David Creswell, a psychologist at Carnegie Mellon University, has been carefully exploring the health effects of mindfulness, as well as how mindfulness may work. Collaborating with Matthew Lieberman at UCLA, whom you may recall was conducting the fMRI brain research, Creswell showed that people who were more mindful displayed a stronger right prefrontal lobe response when engaging in affect labeling; so more mindful people appeared to show a better ability to manage strong negative emotions. In 2013, Creswell and his colleagues reported that participating in an eight-week mindfulness-based stress reduction course improved mindfulness and enhanced the strength of the brain's emotion regulation capacity. In other words, mindfulness training—likely through the practice of affect labeling—led to a better capacity to manage strong negative emotional states, suggesting that interventions, practice, and other approaches can help us improve this important skill.

Although Creswell and others had noted the parallels between mindfulness and expressive writing, another group provided a new piece to the puzzle. Susan Moore and her colleagues conducted a series of studies testing whether expressive writing could facilitate mindfulness. They found that expressive writing did not reliably improve mindfulness for everyone. Rather, those individuals who demonstrated increased mindfulness across writing sessions were also those who showed improvements in mental health. This provides some hint that perhaps writing "works" when it can enhance or increase one's capacity to be mindful.

Kristin Neff at the University of Texas at Austin and her colleagues have been strong advocates of another related approach—promoting self-compassion. The basic idea is to use writing to explore aspects of themselves or issues they have that people don't feel good about: shame, anger, jealousy, greed, whatever it may be. Although there are many specific approaches, generally the writing is meant to facilitate self-kindness and acceptance, focusing on substituting these feelings for self-anger, self-judgment, and self-criticism, along with emphasizing common humanity—the shared broader human experience—rather than feelings of isolation.

Many approaches to self-compassion arise from Buddhist traditions or perspectives, so they may also include efforts to promote mindfulness in ways similar to those discussed above. Mark Leary at Duke University published an impressive series of studies in 2007 demonstrating that naturally occurring levels of self-compassion were related to positive emotional, cognitive, and social processes. At present there is a small but growing research base suggesting that self-compassion interventions can promote positive outcomes, although most involve broader mindfulness-based self-compassion training rather than more narrowly focused self-compassion expressive writing exercises.

When We Can't Simply Shake It Off

Traumatic and other stressful experiences alter the ways we normally think. During most days, we can escape unwanted thoughts by engaging in mindless or low-level thinking. Although low-level thinking may make us unhealthy and even slightly dim-witted, it allows us to screen out feelings of anxiety and pain. As we have seen, it is fairly easy to adopt low-level thinking strategies in the daytime—jogging, drinking, or immersing ourselves in mindless tasks. However, other times we are unable to shake off those unwanted thoughts. Some days we feel a lack of energy, have no desire to do anything, and are left feeling alone with our thoughts—we feel depressed.

It's important to acknowledge that some people can shake off anxiety and other negative emotions much more easily than others. In some cases, this is the result of inherited traits from our parents, particularly difficult childhoods, or other circumstances beyond our control. Over the last decade, for example, studies have suggested that anxiety-prone individuals are more prone to interpret the world in threatening ways than are their less anxious peers.

There is, however, some good news for people who are more anxiety or depression prone. Many expressive writing interventions have been developed to target *just that*. As we noted in Chapter 4, there are relatively few studies that have directly tested expressive writing for major depression or anxiety. An alternative approach is to target individuals who are *at risk* for depression and anxiety. One study, for example, focused on college students who were all prone to depression. Those who benefited most later were those who brooded less. Writing helped them to change the ways they were thinking about their world—perhaps staving off periods of anxiety or depression in the future.

If You Plan to Think Well Tomorrow, You'd Better Get a Good Night's Sleep—or Else

A hallmark of anxiety and depression is insomnia—the inability to sleep.

You lie in bed, partially exhausted, partially tense. You may briefly think about a relationship problem, and then what you need to do tomorrow, and why the room temperature isn't right, and what you should have done yesterday, and back to the relationship problem, and, my God, if you don't fall asleep within 10 minutes you will be exhausted tomorrow. Your thoughts change direction at a furious pace. In the darkness of your room, there are no distractions. Just you—and your thoughts gone wild.

"If there could just be some way to suck out all of these thoughts from my brain," Jamie pondered in the middle of a sleepless night years ago. "Some kind of thought extractor that serves as a psychic vacuum cleaner." Perhaps it was the vacuum cleaner analogy, but it occurred to him that perhaps having people talk into a microphone about their thoughts and feelings could somehow clean out their minds. Their unwanted thoughts would be sucked from their brains into the tape recorder.

Given that he couldn't sleep, Jamie decided to try it. He quietly got up, found a tape recorder, and lay down on the couch in the living room. With his eyes shut and the tape recorder going, he quietly talked about his thoughts and feelings as they occurred to him in a stream-of-consciousness manner. Within 10 minutes, he was sound asleep.

Others have continued to explore the value of disclosure (typically writing or talking) in improving sleep. In a study on poor sleepers, people were asked to write either about worries and concerns or about hobbies. The group that had to write about worries and concerns reported falling asleep more quickly than the hobby or control group. A host of other studies have found that expressive writing before going to bed reduces ruminative thoughts and improves sleep along multiple dimensions.

Why are we telling you this about sleep in a chapter on thinking patterns? In the last decade, scientists across several disciplines are finally starting to realize that sleep quality has profound effects on human functioning. We've known for generations that one of the best markers of depression was disruptions in sleep. We now know that

sleep problems are linked to a variety of major physical health problems and even specifically to problems with the immune system. Similarly, poor sleep is associated with cognitive problems such as poor
memory, difficulty paying attention, accident proneness, and (starting
to sound familiar?) other issues that are similar to mindlessness.

Across multiple studies, one effect of expressive writing (and
some other forms of disclosure) is that it helps to quiet the mind. At
no time could this be more important than when we are trying to get
to sleep.

Final Thoughts on Managing Your Thoughts

We are often surprisingly ignorant of our needs, motivations, and conflicts. When out of control, anxious, or upset, we naturally change our
thinking style. Although low-level thinking can reduce our pain, it
can also narrow our thinking to such an extent that we fail to see that
something is the matter. We can then become the central feature of
our self-constructed paradox: if we naturally escape from the knowledge that something is wrong, how can we ever know about it? How
can we ever hope to control our problem or change our lives?

The answer to the paradox can be deduced from our own behaviors. We should be sensitive to changes in our health, sleep patterns,
and dreams. If we become sick, our illness may reflect some random
virus. But it could also signal a significant stressor that we may be
actively not thinking about. Similarly, sleep problems and major
changes in the content or vividness of dreams can serve as important
bellwethers of our psychological health. Once aware of the warning
signs, we can adjust our thinking levels accordingly.

By now, it should be clear that there are several facets to understanding and coping with unwanted thoughts. Having recurring
thoughts about traumas or other upsetting images is a stressful burden. All of us have had thoughts such as these on occasion. We can
deal with unpleasant thoughts in a variety of ways, many of which
are successful in the short run. Fewer strategies, however, neutralize
unwanted thoughts over the long run.

If you are plagued with unwanted thoughts, remember first that
they are only thoughts. Accept them as your thoughts rather than try
to fight them. One way to cope with thoughts such as these is to write
about them in a self-reflective and emotional manner. What are those

unpleasant thoughts? How do they make you feel? Why? Remember that self-reflection will work far better than wishful thinking in your writing. If you are obsessed with someone's death, for example, wishing he were alive will probably upset you all the more. If you are angry at someone, writing about getting even with her or wishing for her demise will likely exacerbate rather than diminish your ire.

Finally, be attentive to the ways you deal with unwanted thoughts. Low-level thinking, compulsive behaviors, and other distraction strategies can be effective in the short run. Indeed, many stressors we face—such as uncontrollable or unpredictable noises—will go away no matter what we do and will bother us less in a low-level thinking mode. However, if you find that you are now living in a low-level mode to avoid threatening thoughts, it might be time to stand back and reevaluate your coping style.

CHAPTER 7

To Speed Up or Slow Down?

HOW PEOPLE DIFFER IN COPING
WITH TRAUMA

Why do some people deal with major upheavals better than others? What is the secret to healthy coping? We know, for example, that people with supportive social networks weather upheavals better than others. Beyond basic genetic predispositions, do some people adopt certain coping strategies that allow them to move past an upheaval more efficiently? If such coping strategies exist, can they be trained? If such techniques are available, how do they work?

Imagine watching a late-night television commercial. This one would have a fast-talking actor with an insincere look of concern on his face:

> "Hi, folks. Are you out of sorts because your best friend died? Gloomy because your spouse left you for the next-door neighbor? Or just plain down in the dumps because you were fired from your job and face bankruptcy? No problem, folks. For only $49.95, you can get the Power Grieving Solution. In just seven days, you can come to terms with death, separation, or other disaster and start living again. Forget about that old friend, spouse, or job. Get the hassle of grieving over within one week or your money back."

In our culture, we are obsessed with speed and power. We become impatient with the natural pace of things. We can send our two-year-olds to schools to get them to read, swim, or play the piano. Our cars can go much faster than anyone is allowed to drive. Our modern kitchens are equipped with appliances that allow us to prepare and clean up after a meal in record time. We have speed reading, power talking, mind power, and power leadership seminars. We need to suck in our guts and power through lunch, business meetings, and hardships.

Are we ready for Power Grieving™?

There is something both horrifying and fascinating about this idea. Like teaching a two-year-old to read, accelerating the grieving process is toying with the natural order of things. On the other hand, the prolonged pain associated with losing a loved one or dealing with numerous other traumas is often overwhelming. Any techniques that could temper the pain would be welcome by most of us.

Before we contemplate fiddling with the coping process, it's important to consider how coping normally progresses in the real world.

The Natural Sequence of Coping

Sadly, after car and other accidents, suicide is the leading cause of death among adolescents and young adults. Several years ago, a college freshman who attended one of our universities committed suicide by hanging himself in his dormitory room. The student, Darryl, was quiet but well liked. In interviews with other students on his hall, it was striking how differently his friends reacted to the news.

Darryl's next-door neighbor, Newt, for example, was genuinely sorry to learn about the suicide. He talked about it openly and nondefensively. The death, however, didn't appear to affect his behavior in any tangible way. Indeed, he was remarkably well adjusted and happy despite the death. Two months after the death, Newt discussed his reactions:

> It just didn't affect me. Darryl was a great guy and I'm happy that I got to know him. I wish he hadn't killed himself, but he did. Life goes on and sometimes there's no value in looking back.

Contrast Newt's response with that of another hallmate, Omar, who had spoken to Darryl only a few times during the entire school year. The day after the suicide, Omar talked nonstop for an hour and a half. At that point, his emotions vacillated between despair and anger.

His anger was alternately aimed at himself for not seeing signs that Darryl was suicidal and at Darryl himself. Two months later, Omar was still grieving Darryl's death:

At first, I kept thinking "if only I had known." If only I had said something to him or gone by his room that day. Maybe it wouldn't have mattered. It has been hard for me to accept that he died in this building. He did, though. It has been hard in general, but I am slowly coming around. This is the closest I have ever been to death and it scares me. Darryl has caused me to rethink what I want out of life. I hardly even knew Darryl but he has changed me more than anyone since I came to college.

Omar's reactions, unlike Newt's, evolved over time. Whereas Newt appeared to have come to terms with the death almost immediately, Omar was just beginning to move past Darryl's suicide. Whereas Omar's grieving progressed and evolved over time, Newt's seemed to reflect his natural orientation toward life and death. Do most people typically go through a series of stages in coping with traumas, or do they usually have a set grieving style similar to Newt's? Is one approach better or healthier than another?

A Brief History of Coping with Trauma

One of the most impactful books on coping with death, entitled *On Death and Dying,* was published in 1969 by Elisabeth Kübler-Ross. In her book, Kübler-Ross suggested that once people learned they were dying from a terminal disease, they progressed through a series of well-defined stages. Based on hundreds of interviews with terminally ill patients, Kübler-Ross isolated five distinct coping stages: denial, anger, bargaining, depression, and acceptance. Since her original book, others have applied the same stages to people who have had to deal with the death of others, divorce, rape, and other traumas.

The original conception of stages in coping was novel and, in many ways, helpful. It helped explain why people, on learning that they had a life-threatening disease such as cancer, behaved in such different ways. Nurses who work with cancer patients report that more than half of their patients do, in fact, exhibit one or more of the stages suggested by Kübler-Ross at various points during the course of their disease. Some deny either the diagnosis or its fatal implications. Others fly into a rage, threatening to sue the clinic or former employers who may have put them in offices that exposed them to asbestos or other carcinogenic agents. A number of forms of bargaining can also be seen. Some become deeply religious, implicitly hoping that now that their soul has been saved, their body will be spared. Depression, not surprisingly, can be an intermittent problem for many people with advanced cancer. Acceptance refers to the fundamental understanding that death will occur. Once patients accept the fact of their own impending death, they often exhibit a sense of peace and contentment.

The major difficulty with Kübler-Ross's stage models, however, is that not everyone goes through all or even most of the stages that were originally posited. In fact, it is common for a person to bounce from one stage, such as anger, to another, such as acceptance, and then back to anger again. Researchers often find Kübler-Ross's model frustrating, since it doesn't (and cannot) predict or explain who will progress through which stages. Many counselors and therapists have also become disillusioned because it fails to specify how to get patients to the acceptance phase or otherwise facilitate their adjustment. For example, should a terminally ill cancer patient who is angry about his or her diagnosis be encouraged to move on to bargaining or getting depressed?

Despite the lingering popularity of Kübler-Ross's model, most researchers have moved on. Other, simpler stage models have been tested with limited success. For example, Mardi Horowitz, who studies individuals who have faced major traumas such as rape, has proposed that people often go through three general stages: denial, working through, and completion. The goal of therapy, in Horowitz's view, is to aid in the working-through phase so that completion (also called assimilation, reflecting a sense of acceptance or understanding) is attained.

Even a three-phase model of coping doesn't satisfy most therapists and researchers because people rarely react to traumatic events in identical ways. Equally puzzling is that any given therapy may be beneficial for some, ineffective for others, and, for a small subset, sometimes harmful.

Standing back and looking at the growing literature on coping, a number of basic principles seem to be emerging:

- Human beings are amazingly resilient. The majority of people cope well with massive upheavals in their lives.
- Intensive therapy or counseling in the hours and days after a massive upheaval is typically *not* beneficial. In fact, there is some evidence that pushing people to talk about their feelings too much in the immediate aftermath of a trauma may increase the likelihood of long-term emotional problems.
- Some traumas require different coping strategies than others. What may be beneficial for one type of upheaval may not be helpful for another.
- There are large differences in the ways people cope with traumas. People are often their own best counselors.

The Resilience of People

Some people are deeply scarred after experiencing a horrible event such as rape, seeing or being the victim of violence, or surviving a major car accident. A common diagnosis following such an event is PTSD. People suffering from PTSD may experience unwanted thoughts, images, or dreams of the upheaval. They try to avoid the memories of the event by not talking about it or not seeing people or places that might remind them of what happened. It is common for PTSD sufferers to begin using drugs or alcohol to escape the memories and feelings. They often feel alienated, anxious, or depressed and have trouble working, focusing their attention, and spending time with other people. Make no mistake. PTSD is a real phenomenon that can be devastating.

If you read the popular press—or even psychology journals—you might conclude that PTSD and other mental and physical health problems are the standard responses to all large traumas. Surprisingly, the opposite is true. Most people deal with traumatic experiences quite well with no major changes in their mental or physical health. In a series of classic articles, Roxane Silver from the University of California at Irvine and Camille Wortman from Stony Brook University summarized a large number of studies indicating that the majority of people who have faced the death of a spouse or child did *not* experience intense anxiety, depression, or grief that lasted for months or years. Similarly, approximately two-thirds of soldiers who have fought in horrific battles or war zones never show any evidence of PTSD. Once again, the majority of people who have survived major motor vehicle accidents or witnessed tragic airplane accidents did not experience depression or PTSD in the months after their experiences. Across several studies, up to 80 percent of rape survivors did not show substantial and sustained symptoms of PTSD.

This is not to say that people who have experienced these horrible events did not feel deeply upset, grieve, cry, or need the comfort of others. Most *were* profoundly upset. But in the days, weeks, and months that followed, most coped well. Some talked a great deal to their friends. Others spent time alone. Yet others immediately returned to their everyday lives seemingly unscathed.

This is an important point. If you have a friend who has experienced an unimaginable trauma and, a few days later, he seems to be relatively happy and behaving normally, he may be relatively happy and behaving normally. It is entirely possible that he is not repressing his feelings or seething with hidden grief or rage.

Psychotherapy Is Often Not Needed after a Traumatic Experience

Mental health workers are generally very good, caring people. After an earthquake or tornado or something like the September 11, 2001, attacks in New York City, they rush in to help people cope with the experience. After school suicides or shootings, grief counselors are among the first to talk with students and staff. The underlying assumption is that people are fragile and they need support from professionals.

Both of us have long been interested in how people respond to, and cope with, natural and man-made disasters. For example, Jamie has studied people's reactions to the Mt. St. Helens volcano eruption in 1981, the Loma Prieta earthquake in 1989, the U.S. reaction to the outbreak of the Persian Gulf War in 1991, the September 11th attacks, and other incidents. He has also been interested in more common events—a neighborhood murder, the unexpected death of friends, a crime spree that terrorized a community.

Across all large- and small-scale upheavals he studied, people came together. A natural response to a terrible experience is to talk with others. In the aftermath of the Mt. St. Helens eruption, the city of Yakima, Washington, was buried under up to four inches of ash. It terrified many people and caused huge disruptions. Ironically, in interviews of people a month later, most remarked that the eruption brought the community together. It gave them the opportunity to meet neighbors they didn't know they had.

On the afternoon of September 11th, a small army of psychotherapists went to downtown Manhattan to provide free therapy. No one was interested. One of our good psychologist friends was there to provide support, and she noted that the only people she spoke with were other psychologists. For most major upheavals in our lives, we have existing social networks to support us. In other words, most people probably don't need therapy after a trauma because they have their own friends and acquaintances to do the therapeutic work.

A more substantial question concerns the need for therapy in the first hours or days after a traumatic experience. We know that in the medical field emergency medicine has developed groundbreaking procedures to save lives. No such advances have been made in the mental health field. In fact, attempts to develop emergency therapeutic care for mental health have met with many unforeseen problems.

One of the bigger controversies in the helping profession grew out of an intervention called critical incident stress debriefing, or CISD. In the 1970s, Jeff Mitchell was working as a paramedic who supported firefighters, police, and other rescue workers in responding to health emergencies, accidents, suicides, and other often gory and tragic events. Jeff noticed that a number of the emergency workers never talked about the events and many were depressed, moody, and suffered from a range of personal problems the longer they worked on the job. With no formal psychological training, he developed a brief program to aid rescue workers soon after an upsetting event. The basic idea was to get the rescue workers together within 24 hours of the event and have them share their personal feelings and experiences about the event.

The debriefing idea made good sense. It was the first program of its kind, and the idea quickly caught on. In fact, within a few years, the CISD movement was adopted by governmental agencies across the world. Armies of people visited Mitchell's company in Maryland to be trained in the procedure. Firefighting and police departments as well as multiple agencies within the U.S. government all had people trained in, and ready to deliver, the CISD method.

The only problem is that no one had ever done any serious scientific studies to see if CISD worked. It *sounded* good. It *should* have worked. But the first independent studies suggested that it didn't work. In fact, several researchers began to warn that debriefing too soon after a trauma might actually be harmful for some people. In hindsight, parts of the CISD strategy probably were beneficial. But the debriefing component—where people were actively encouraged to express their emotions and vulnerabilities, often in the presence of their superiors, peers, and/or subordinates—was problematic.

Immediately after a traumatic experience, most people are somewhat stunned—almost in a state of shock. They are overwhelmed with their own emotions and the emotions of others. A massive upheaval can touch every part of their lives. To sort out the complexity of the experience can take days or weeks. People who are already emotionally and cognitively overloaded benefit from less information rather than more information. In short, pressing people to experience more emotions in the hours or days after a major experience can be overwhelming and likely unhelpful.

If emotional debriefing immediately after a trauma doesn't work, what about expressive writing? It's the same problem. Pushing people to write about a major emotional experience immediately after it has occurred has not been found to be helpful.

What *does* work after a traumatic experience? How can you help a close friend in the aftermath of something horrible? Currently, the common wisdom among PTSD experts is to provide safety (both physical and psychological), to answer questions that the traumatized person is asking, and to be a good listener (typically this means being supportive and nonjudgmental). Some people really do benefit from talking or writing. In that case, let them talk or write. Some want to play video games to distract themselves. Encourage them to play video games. Others want to sit alone and cry. That's fine too.

This advice is also relevant to you if something traumatic befalls you. There is no "official" way to cope with a trauma. Follow your own instincts. In most cases, your friends will be understanding of your choices. If you have some friends who are pushing you to do things you don't want to do, giving you advice you don't want to hear, or forcing you to eat another turkey casserole dish that you can't stand, just thank them (they likely mean well) and ask them to give you a bit of time by yourself.

The Differences among Traumas:
The Special Case of Bereavement

The first edition of this book was published in 1990. At the time, most social scientists assumed that the death of a loved one was similar to other major upheavals in life. It was an emotional event, it touched most parts of a person's life, it was personal. Although no expressive writing studies had been conducted on people who had experienced the death of someone close, it was assumed that writing would be beneficial. Why wouldn't it?

About the same time, Margaret and Wolfgang Stroebe started a series of large projects in Tübingen, Germany, studying people whose spouses had died within the previous year. They are superb scientists, and their studies involved large groups of adults and were always impeccably designed. In one writing study, over 120 widowed participants were randomly assigned to write about the death of their spouse in one of three ways or asked to simply complete questionnaires. One group in particular was encouraged to write about their thoughts and feelings about the death.

In contrast to earlier studies on expressive writing, the authors found no effect of writing. In an impressive overview of the bereavement literature in 2007, the Stroebes summarized 20 experiments on a variety of grief-related interventions on recently bereaved adults. The interventions included standard grief counseling, forms of cognitive-behavioral therapy, and expressive writing. Virtually none of the interventions had any mental or physical health benefits. Although there were typically no adverse responses to any of the interventions, most of the common therapeutic approaches that psychologists and social workers had always believed in simply had no effect. For writing researchers, these patterns were disappointing.

But wait. There might be hope after all. All of the early bereavement studies were "outreaching" studies. An outreaching study is one where investigators contact a large group of people who have faced the death of a spouse. That is, the surviving spouse simply responds to a request to participate in an experiment. Sixteen of the original bereaved studies that failed to show beneficial effects were all outreaching studies.

Most of the recent—and successful—bereavement experiments relied on "inreaching" methodologies. An inreaching study uses bereaved people who have contacted counselors or group therapy experts on their own because they are having trouble adjusting. In other words, those who know they are having problems and are open to seeking and receiving help actually benefit from grief interventions and, presumably, from expressive writing.

Another interesting twist in grief intervention work has also emerged. Methods such as expressive writing have now shown some hints that they may be beneficial for traumatic grief cases. Traumatic grief involves cases where the death of the loved one was completely unexpected—often because of an accident, suicide, or murder. Similarly, in situations of complicated or chronic grief, writing or other grief interventions can be helpful. Complicated grief occurs when the death was confounded with other terrible experiences—for example, where a spouse dies and it is discovered that there are huge debts because of an unknown gambling problem, resulting in the loss of the surviving spouse's home. In addition, people diagnosed with chronic grief tend to see the world as one where the spouse's death simply made everything in their lives worse.

Let's stand back a moment and think about the pattern of effects. Grief interventions, including expressive writing, seem to work only if the bereavement is traumatic or complicated. Simple, uncomplicated grief—the kind most of us experience when dealing with the loss of a parent, close friend, or even a pet—can be intermittently powerful and painful for weeks, months, or years. Why can't therapeutic interventions lessen the pain?

Several bereavement scholars point to the central difference between the loss of a loved one and other traumas we might experience. Being a victim of a horrible assault can shatter a person's view about the predictability of the world. A humiliating failure can undermine one's sense of efficacy and destroy one's friendship circle. But the death of a loved one gets at the very essence of our bonds with other people. Our connections to our parents, our spouse, our children are primitive and partially define who we are.

The links between social and emotional attachment and grief have been discussed since John Bowlby first introduced the concept of the attachment bond between parent and child in the mid-20th century. Researchers are now beginning to find that people with secure attachments to their parents are able to cope better with the loss of a parent than those with more anxious attachments. The links we established with our parents when we were young children, it is argued, define how we hold on to (and let go of) all of our social bonds.

Understand Your Attachment Style

There are many different ways to identify your attachment style, some of which are available online. The following sites provide information, including a relatively short quiz that not only helps determine your attachment style but will also help explain what the different aspects of attachment mean and how they may be impacting your relationships.

> www.web-research-design.net/cgi-bin/crq/crq.pl
> www.psychologytoday.com/basics/attachment
> www.psychalive.org/what-is-your-attachment-style
> http://psychology.about.com/od/loveandattraction/ss/
>   attachmentstyle.htm

Whereas most traumas and trauma therapies are based on repairing people's self- and worldviews, bereavement and grief involve coming to terms with the permanent loss of another person and the role that person played.

Love and Grief: A Temporal Theory

We have yet to have a distraught person come into our offices and ask, "I am madly in love. When can I expect these feelings to go away?" As anyone who has been in love knows, the quality of love changes over time. Love can be passionate, delicate, or deep and abiding. Grief, too, changes in its intensity and tenor. There exists a recurring pattern in the evolution of powerful emotions. Rather than a gradual diminution of intense feelings over time, significant emotional states seem to transform themselves in stages. Although there are differences from person to person, most overpowering feeling states exhibit three distinct stages over a year and a half: intensity, plateau, and assimilation.

For both love and grief, people first enter a stage of intense emotional activation, which lasts between four and six months. During the intensity stage, individuals constantly think about their new or departed lover. At about six months, people move to a relatively constant plateau of getting on with life. The plateau period, which lasts about a year, is characterized by a generally pleasant (in the case of love) or unpleasant (grief) mood state. Although people think about their new or departed love many times each day, the thoughts are more reflective and less emotionally charged. Around a year and a half after the entire process began, most people have assimilated or come to terms with the love or death. In the assimilation stage, passionate love is replaced by an enduring, loving friendship. In the place of intense grief come fond memories and new experiences.

Julie versus Ellen: A Comparison of Diaries

Over the years, several people have generously allowed us to read and study their personal diaries. Particularly interesting are the diaries of people who appear to be exceptionally healthy and well adjusted. Two diaries stand out. The first was written by a 26-year-old woman named Julie who had kept a diary since she was only 10. When she was 22, she fell deeply in love with Charles. The second diary was written by Ellen, who, at the age of 60, unexpectedly lost John, her husband of 40 years, to a heart attack. Five years after John's death she remarried and flourished.

The intensity stage is easiest to identify. During the first four to six months, lovers and grievers are consumed with new emotions and recurring thoughts. The following diary entries were written two weeks after Julie's first date with Charles and, for Ellen, two weeks after the death of John.

> JULIE: *I think I am in love! I honestly have never felt this way before about anyone—I **love** being with Charles and my God he occupies my every thought. This weekend we were together the whole time . . . I feel like I'm walking on clouds. It's the best!*

> ELLEN: *Two weeks today. It's like yesterday and like forever. I stroked his dear dead face and said, "Goodnight, sweet prince." And my beautiful life ended.*

Three months later, both women were still in a stage of emotional intensity. Both diaries, however, indicate that the women were also beginning to think of other things. Their respective feelings of joy and grief, however, were dominant.

JULIE: *The trip to California with Charles! It was the best trip ever. Since then we have talked so much and written many a letter back and forth. I've never felt like this before—it's a new one for me, that's for sure.*

ELLEN: *Three months and where am I? I play foolish games. His shaving glasses are still on the shaving mirror. I cry when I see dust on them, but I can't throw them away . . . I still have aching memories of his death and of sad days in Spain. I wish he hadn't suffered.*

Soon after these entries, the tenor of the emotions changed, suggesting that both women had entered the plateau phase. Julie, although she frequently refers to Charles, devotes much of her writing to problems at work or telephone conversations with her parents. Charles's presence, however, is always felt. Four months after the death of Bob, Ellen stopped writing in her diary for almost eight months. The reason, she said, was that she was trying to get on with life. Interestingly, it was during this period that Ellen volunteered to help a bereavement counselor write manuals on coping with death.

The following entry by Julie was written seven months after her first date with Charles. The entries for the previous week had been devoted to topics other than Charles.

Last night Charles and I had another talk. I am convinced that we will end up together later in life. I am in love with him and he knows I am. It's very special. Sometimes I really do get scared about the future. I think we will be fine—it's just that I have never been in love before and here we are talking about the future. I'm learning a lot from this relationship—both about him and myself.

A little after one year, both Julie and Ellen exhibit signs of standing back and analyzing their situations. In Julie's situation, the mad passion is no longer ever present. For Ellen, there has been a sharp drop in the intense grief she had been feeling in the four months after John's death.

JULIE: *What is he thinking? It's like I want to jump inside his mind and know each thing that goes through his head. When we aren't hand in hand or not smiling I think that something's wrong.* **Try reality***, Julie.*

Couples aren't constantly smiling—starry eyed . . . Oh, I do feel good about being with him. I feel that we are very close. Closer than I've ever been with anyone. But I do make it difficult for people to get to know me.

ELLEN: *It's been a year of selfishness. I've mainly thought of my own comfort, my own needs. I suppose it's time now to broaden my outlook and I hope this will come, in time, but I still have hangups that put obstacles in my way. The longing is gone, I guess. He's gone, and he'll never come back to me. Oh, but I miss him so . . . It's better and I think it will continue to get even better. I really rejoice to see how the children and I have moved on . . . and that's as it should be.*

Signs of the assimilation stage were apparent a few months later. Almost exactly a year and a half after their first date, Julie and Charles moved in together. Julie's journal entries became much more sporadic. When Charles was mentioned, it was usually in the context of a disagreement or noting the differences in their personalities. Otherwise, her writing reflected a union between them. Many of her experiences were now expressed in the first-person plural "we" as their shared experiences: "We went camping and we felt so thrilled by the fresh air."

A year and a half after John's death, Ellen took on a new job, sold her house, and moved into an apartment. She stopped her diary writing altogether. In talking about her diary, Ellen noted that she "just got stronger" and didn't need to write any longer. She knew that John would have wanted it as much as she needed it.

The temporal model can be quite useful in evaluating people's reactions to both positive and negative events, although it should not be applied rigidly. The transition points at 6 and 18 months vary considerably depending on several factors. For completely new, unique, and overpowering life events, the 6- and 18-month time periods appear to serve as useful guideposts that describe typical timelines for understanding the reactions of about half of all people. Yet with this said, these times can fluctuate one way or another by several months depending on other events that may occur in the interim. The time periods are usually much shorter for people who have been passionately in love before (in the case of understanding love) or for those who have suffered another major loss (in the case of grief).

Is Power Grieving™ or, Perhaps, Power Coping™ in Our Future?

It's fairly clear that there is no way to speed up normal, uncomplicated grief. In the future, we will all face personal losses due to death. For some, talking about the loss might be helpful. For others, simply getting on with life might be best. In the foreseeable future, no one-size-fits-all therapy is on the horizon.

How about power coping? Are there ways to accelerate the ways we get over emotional upheavals? For this, there might be more promise.

Easing the College Transition

Several years ago, Jamie and several of his students sought to learn whether it would be possible to speed up the adjustment time of first-year college students. Although not typically a traumatic experience, leaving home and moving into a college dormitory around age 18 is a major upheaval for most students. The transition to college involves leaving family and friends, and changing roles within their families and within society in general. There are often substantial economic burdens on top of learning to live in a completely new environment. It is well established that the transition to college is associated with high levels of loneliness, depression, and increased physical and psychological health problems. Further, new social pressures often make it difficult for the new students to be open and honest with their peers.

An illustration of the conflicts felt by many beginning students can be seen in the following writing sample. The author, a woman who had come to college only a month earlier, wrote this passage as a participant in one of our studies:

> I believed college was going to be a fun, exciting experience. Now that I'm here though, I find it's not all that way. This is the first time I've been away from home, and although I've met a lot of new friends, sometimes I feel like I am all alone, that I am living with a bunch of strangers and no one really knows who I am or what I am about. Living in my dorm is fun, but I feel like I always have to act like someone I'm really not just so people will like me. At home, I would get in bad moods and be bitchy to

my family, but I feel I cannot do that here because then everyone always
says you're a bitch and talks behind your back.

In a test to see if it was possible to accelerate people's adjustment
to college, about 130 entering freshmen were asked to write either
about superficial topics or about their deepest thoughts and feelings
about coming to college. Those in the expressive writing condition
were told:

> "For each of the writing sessions, I want you to let go and write about
> your very deepest thoughts and feelings about coming to college. . . .
> In your writing, you might want to write about your emotions and
> thoughts about leaving your friends or parents, about issues of adjusting
> to the various aspects of college . . . or even about your feelings of who
> you are or what you want to become."

As a test of coping acceleration, students were run in one of four
waves. The first wave of 33 students participated during the first week
of classes in early September. The next wave wrote during the first
week of October; wave three close to the beginning of November;
wave four during the first week of December. The purpose of running
people in waves was to see if adjustment to college could be sped up.
If the "power coping" concept was valid, there would be health and
psychological benefits for wave-one participants equivalent to those of
wave four.

Power coping worked. Whenever people wrote about coming
to college—whether it was the first week of classes or three months
later—visits to the doctor for illnesses dropped afterward. People who
wrote about superficial topics, in a pattern consistent with what you
see from college students more generally, demonstrated a gradual
increase in physician visits over the course of the first semester.

A second phenomenon of interest concerned the long-term health
benefits of writing. In general, writing about coming to college promoted health for a little over four months. By the fifth month after
writing, however, students who had written about their thoughts
and feelings were getting as sick as everyone else; in other words, the
beneficial effects appeared to have worn off. Writing about upsetting
experiences for three days, then, does not bring about permanent
health improvements.

Like the students in this study, both of us had some ambivalence about our first year in college. Although exhilarated by our new free-doms, we also had periods of feeling lonely, depressed, and incompe-tent. However, whenever people asked us how we were liking college, we would immediately paint forced grins on our faces and remark that college was wonderful, great, *really* terrific. Perhaps, had we been participants in our own experiments back then, we would have been a little more honest with ourselves and others about the complicated feelings surrounding college.

Caveat Emptor

Confronting ongoing crises appears to promote long-term health and adjustment. In this experiment, the coping process was accelerated for many of the participants. Keep in mind, however, that we are dealing with statistics—benefits were seen overall, or on average, for the groups of students participating in the study. Not everyone was helped. In terms of illness measures, for example, most people did not change in their physician visits from before to after writing. Overall, about 11 percent of the participants who wrote about college got sicker after participating in the study compared with 39 percent of the stu-dents who wrote about trivial topics. Extrapolating across our various measures, the experiment probably resulted in a real improvement in physical and psychological health for 20 to 30 percent of the partici-pants. Put more cynically, the experiment did not affect the majority of students one way or the other. As we noted earlier, Camille Wort-man and Roxane Silver conclude from their projects that as many as half of all people naturally cope fairly well, even with major traumas. It is entirely possible that these roll-with-the-punches individuals are not helped significantly by writing about crises.

Not all people roll with the punches, however. Although writ-ing about ongoing crises is clearly helpful for many, the effect is nei-ther instantaneous nor permanent. In the minutes immediately after writing about coming to college, many participants felt less happy, more homesick, and more anxious about college in general—similar to immediate responses we see to expressive writing in other contexts. Although health improvements were apparent soon after writing, the effects lasted only about four months.

As we have noted before, neither writing about nor confronting upsetting experiences is a panacea that will work for all people all the time. Yet, across thousands of people in dozens of different experiments, there is clearly a net positive effect. If you are currently facing a major crisis in your life, don't expect that writing will make your life wonderful. The magical idea of "power coping" is a misnomer in that most crises take a long time to overcome and may involve a difficult process. All that these experiments promise is that, for many people, writing can reduce the grieving time and enhance adjustment and well-being. Finally, remember that this early project focused on one particular type of crisis: the transition to college. In the grand scheme of traumas, going to college is significant but very likely not catastrophic.

Final Thoughts and Some Important Lessons about Coping

It appears to be the case that the coping process can be accelerated. But there are some very real qualifications to this statement. Always read the fine print when something sounds too good to be true. Herewith the fine print:

• *Many people naturally cope well with traumas.* Not everyone progresses through stages in grieving or coping. In fact, as many as half of all adults who face some serious traumatic experiences (divorce, the loss of a loved one, torture, or some other catastrophe) may not exhibit any major signs of depression or anxiety. Almost by definition, then, a substantial number of people may not benefit from attempts to influence their coping strategies.

It is critical to appreciate the large differences among people in coping with trauma. For example, if you see someone who, after suffering a major trauma, appears to be relatively normal, happy, and nondefensive, it is entirely possible that the person really is doing just fine. Never discount that many people do, in fact, roll with the punches.

Conversely, at least 20 percent of the population *does* experience major depression, anxiety, or other signs of grief following a trauma. Among these people, coping strategies will also vary tremendously—often in unpredictable ways. Denial, anger, low-level thinking, and other defense mechanisms may occur at random intervals or even in sequence. Among those who do exhibit signs of grief, writing or talking about the experience is likely to help.

• *The degree to which coping can be accelerated is limited.* Coming to terms with any major upheaval takes time. No known procedure can help you overcome a significant personal loss overnight. If your lover left you yesterday, for example, writing about it may shorten the time that you suffer from, say, five months to three months. But then, no one knows. For some people, writing or talking about a trauma can make a dramatic difference; for others it may have no effect whatsoever.

By the same token, the benefits of writing or talking about a trauma may be temporary. The coming-to-college study indicated that the health benefits lasted about four months. Even now, largely due to the complexities and costs of following research participants over long periods of time, very few studies have examined health effects over periods longer than six months.

• *Potential problems if you are still in the midst of a crisis.* If you are currently in the middle of a divorce, someone close to you has just died, or you have suffered some other major trauma quite recently, writing or talking about your experience may not be helpful. If you want to write, then do so. But do not push yourself (or anyone else). You can do deep emotional processing about the experience in the future. You might even find that exercising, playing video games, or watching TV is more therapeutic for now.

A related issue about ongoing crises is that, by their very nature, new upsetting events may still be in store for you. If, for example, you are in the middle of a divorce, writing about it may help you come to terms with being alone. It may not prepare you for a future ugly trial, vicious rumors, or receiving the final divorce papers in the mail.

• *And the usual admonitions.* The ways you write or talk about upsetting experiences are important. In your writing, explore your deepest thoughts and feelings in a self-reflective way. Set aside a specific time and location to write continuously. If you talk to someone else, it helps if the person is objective and not personally involved. Don't be surprised if you feel somewhat sad or depressed immediately after writing. The work of self-reflection can sometimes be painful even if the benefits down the line are clear. We provide more details on how to write effectively in Chapter 10.

CHAPTER 8

"I'm Here for You . . . or Am I?"

THE AUDIENCE ON THE OTHER END OF OUR WORDS

Most individual traumas have social components. Even if they are not caused by other people, we often turn to others to cope with them. This inherently social aspect of disclosing traumas has important meaning not only for the people who experience the trauma, but for those who hear about it as well.

Consider the case of Laura, a 35-year-old lawyer. When she was 10 years old, Laura's parents divorced. Two years after the divorce, her mother remarried. Six months after the marriage, Laura's stepfather began to drink heavily. About the time she turned 13, Laura's life changed. Late one night, she awoke to find her drunken stepfather fondling her breasts. Although she slapped him and demanded that he leave, he made light of the situation. This continued off and on until Laura was 15, at which time she left home to live with her aunt. Not until she developed uterine cancer at age 24 did she admit this experience to anyone.

Laura recounted the agony of those two years:

I had always been close to my mother. The divorce had nearly killed her and she was so happy with Jock [the stepfather]. If she had known what Jock was doing to me, it would have broken her heart. I wanted to tell her

so much. Do you know what it is like to be in a family like that? I'd get up
in the morning and Jock and my mother would come down together. He
would smile and be friendly, like nothing had happened. I hated his guts
but could never tell anyone why. Every morning, every evening, every time
I saw that bastard, I felt sick to my stomach. I guess it's not surprising that
I developed an ulcer before my 15th birthday.

Looking back on it all, the very worst thing was that I couldn't talk to
my mother anymore. I had to keep a wall between us. If I wasn't careful,
the wall might crumble and I'd tell her everything. The same was true of
my friends. I'd go out with my girlfriends and we would all giggle about
boys and dating. Their giggles were real, mine weren't. If they had known
what was happening in my bedroom they would have died.

Laura was put into an impossible social bind. Had she told her
mother, there would have been a massive family upheaval. Had Laura
told her friends, her disclosure would have caused an uproar. It was
possible her mother might not have believed her (which often happens when children implicate a family member in sexual abuse). Her
friends may have deserted her. Even the best possible scenario would
have exposed Laura to being stigmatized by some people in her neighborhood or school.

Throughout this book, we have pointed out the dangers of keeping secrets. But we haven't yet acknowledged that people often keep
secrets for very good reasons or in response to tremendous social pressures. One such reason is that revealing deeply personal secrets puts
people at risk of becoming outcasts among their friends. In an important article on the processes surrounding disclosure, Stephenie Chaudoir and Jeff Fisher point to the importance of "stigma management."
The idea is that when we have a potentially threatening secret that
we want to tell others, we gradually let parts of the secret out—little
by little, in small doses. As we do this, we are closely monitoring our
friends to see how they react. If they seem even slightly disturbed,
threatened, or hurt, we back away and alter our story to make it less
threatening. This is done to protect the friendship, and achieved by
keeping the secret.

There is another side to this phenomenon as well—think about
the listener's perspective. It's usually painful to hear someone we
know recount a personal tragedy that he or she has experienced.
We may relish reading about fires, murders, or messy divorces in the
newspaper, but when the same events involve people we care about,

they can be extremely distressing. In fact, if we know that someone has had a particularly troubling experience, many times we might avoid calling, visiting, or even seeing the person. What should we say? Does she want to talk about it? Do I really want to hear about it?

Talking about and Reacting to Trauma: The Loss of a Loved One

The death of a child violates every conception of meaning that we hold about the world. For parents, the mere thought of their children's death inspires nothing short of terror. Several years ago, Jamie was invited to speak to a support group of bereaved parents who had recently faced that ultimate horror. One by one, the parents recounted their experiences of learning of the deaths of their children by murder, suicide, car accidents, and disease. Racial, social class, and religious differences were completely irrelevant. Their bond was a common tragedy.

Because Jamie had been studying the cognitive changes that accompanied tragedies, he had planned to discuss ways to come to terms with death. Given his research, he understood what they must be going through, he assured them. The group sat respectfully listening to the "expert" talk about something he couldn't even fathom. After his brief talk, there was an icy silence in the air.

Finally, a man in the back row raised his hand and said in a gentle voice, "You don't know what we feel—no one can ever know until it happens." Everyone nodded in agreement. "Please, never say that you understand what we are going through because you can't. Some of our friends say the same thing and they don't know what they're talking about."

An honest discussion emerged. Their children's death was beyond description in terms of its impact. What they were least prepared for, however, was their social isolation. Yes, the two or three weeks after the death, their friends had been wonderful—bringing food by the house, offering to help do the shopping, taking care of their other children. But then the phone calls stopped. Their friends and coworkers began to avoid them. Casual conversations became stilted because no one wanted to broach the topic of the death.

One couple tearfully recounted what had happened to them in

the months following the death of their two-year-old son. They were deeply religious, and their entire social life revolved around their small, tightly knit church. In fact, the church had organized several services to pray for their son when he was diagnosed with a terminal liver disease. About a month after their son's death, the couple began to feel ostracized by the minister and other church members. Former close friends no longer sat by them during regular church services. They were no longer invited to informal social gatherings. Whenever they tried to talk about their son's death, people quickly changed the topic of conversation. In the span of a few months, they had lost their son and their entire social support group. Finally, when they hinted to their minister that they might join another church in a neighboring town, he agreed that it "would probably be best for everyone."

The Loss of Social Support after a Loved One Dies

The social problems faced by bereaved parents are readily apparent. The parents desperately want to talk about their loss with others. Their friends, however, find the topic too horrifying and psychologically threatening to even think about. Friends of the grieving parents often deal with the problem by simply avoiding the parents altogether.

The benefit of talking about one's problems is largely dependent on the social response from the audience. A therapist provides a safe environment. Personal relationships with family, spouses, friends, or coworkers may be a different story, as these individuals may typically not respond as we would like them to, and therefore talking to them may do more harm than good. Again, it is important to note that this is not *always* the case. Some evidence suggests that emotional disclosure is not necessary for coping with loss in an adaptive way. Nevertheless, for those who desire or need to express their thoughts or emotions, *not* being able to do so can be a major stressor.

A recent study documents this well. Vanessa Juth and her colleagues assessed the health of over 200 bereaved individuals several years after their loss. Those people who reported feeling the greatest pressure from others to not talk about their loss were the people who reported the most mental and physical health problems. Social constraints are like subtle social handcuffs. Friends of the bereaved people undoubtedly sent out nonverbal signals that said, "Let's not discuss anything emotionally threatening."

The problem of social constraints is made worse by the lack of any clear norms on how to behave. In interviews, friends of people who have faced a trauma fear that, by broaching the topic, they will upset the traumatized person. On numerous occasions, we have heard individuals say, "I didn't want to remind them about it" or "I thought it would be best to try to keep their minds off it," or even, "if they wanted to talk about it, they would have said so." These rationalizations that most of us have used at one time or another may occasionally be true. In all likelihood, however, we usually employ these beliefs so that we won't have to hear about the traumas ourselves.

If a friend of yours has suffered the death of a child or other relative, or faced some other significant trauma, your friend is probably thinking about it a great deal. Don't be hesitant to ask if he or she would like to talk about it. Platitudes such as "You will get over it," "I know just how you feel," or "At least you had some good times together" are usually not helpful. Unless you have dealt with a similar trauma, you probably don't know how your friend feels. For your friend's own good, let him or her talk freely about the loss. Finally, if you have fond memories of your friend's loved one, mention them. Even if the death occurred several years earlier, your friend will be glad that the person's memory lives on.

If you have suffered a loss, many of your friends will not know what to say or how to deal with your feelings. It is easy to interpret your friends' behaviors as being cruel or insensitive, when this probably is not the case. Very often, they would like to talk about the tragedy but don't know how to bring up the subject. In casual conversations, both you and your friend may be thinking about your loss, but neither person says anything. As one person explained, "It is as if there is a giant elephant in the living room and both of us pretend nothing is there." Bereaved parents who have coped well note that they have learned to say something like "Please feel free to talk about it." In other words, the burden of introducing the topic will be on you.

Finally, we strongly recommend support groups. In most cities, there are groups of people who have suffered traumas similar to yours. For the loss of a child, groups such as Compassionate Friends or Bereaved Parents can be invaluable. Similar groups are available for people who have lost a lover, spouse, or family member due to suicide, illness, or other tragedy. Other organizations that focus on specific problems such as drug and alcohol problems, eating disorders, compulsive gambling, smoking, victimization from rape or violence, and spouse or child abuse can be found in most areas of the country. If you are unable to locate a relevant group, contact a United Way office or crisis center in your area. Note that groups such as these encourage conversation among people who have faced similar problems rather than provide therapy or counseling per se.

Marital Problems Resulting from Shared Traumas

In many friendships where one person has experienced a trauma and the other hasn't, the two people are in fundamentally different psychological states. A very different problem occurs when two people have both suffered the same loss. Among parents who have lost a child, the statistics are depressing. In the years afterward, one or both members of the couple have much higher rates of major illness, psychiatric problems, and death rates in general. Although divorce rates may be higher than the national average, these statistics are more controversial. Couples who share other types of traumas, such as financial ruin, the arrest of a child, or even more mild challenges such as moving to a new community are similarly at higher risk for marital problems.

A shared trauma is particularly difficult because neither person is able to provide strong support for the other, since both are grieving. This problem is compounded in that people tend to grieve at their own pace, in their own way. A tragic example of this was evident in an interview with Dolores, a woman who had recently separated from her husband of 18 years following the accidental shooting death of their 14-year-old son seven months earlier:

> Bob [her husband] withdrew the minute he heard about the shooting. He would sit at the supper table and not say a word. I always was crying, wanting to talk about Mikey [the son]. Bob sometimes just got mad at me for talking so much. The more I wanted him to listen, the quieter he got. . . . He didn't touch me. He didn't want anything to do with me. . . . Bob's brother told me that they'd go fishing together and sometimes he would cry like a baby. After Mikey's death, I never saw one tear from him.

Dolores's case raises the issue of the potentially quite different grieving styles of men and women. In recent research, Margaret Stroebe and her colleagues find that it is not uncommon for either the man or the woman to play the role of "the strong one" to help a partner cope. In an in-depth study of over 200 bereaved couples, the research team discovered that this pattern of holding in one's grief to help bolster the other was common among both men and women. What made the study interesting was that this pattern—which they call "partner-oriented self-regulation," or POSR—is ultimately damaging to both partners in the relationship. Couples who rely on POSR ultimately experience much more grief and stress than those where both members of the couple are open and honest with each other about their feelings. Communication, whether by openly expressing emotions or simply by talking, is one of the keys to the survival of a relationship following a shared trauma.

Disclosure and Relationship Trauma

Most long-term intimate relationships undergo periods of stress and upheaval. Financial hardships, job uncertainty, parenting stressors, and marital fidelity issues are some of many factors that can shake partners' sense of stability. Writing about relationship distress and trauma may help couples build a shared way of looking at the world, which boosts intimacy and trust. Studies on expressive writing have been tried with couples dealing with extramarital affairs, often in the form of letter-writing. One approach asks members of a couple to write a letter to the other outlining their thoughts and feelings. Afterward, couples typically exhibit reductions in feelings of distress and depression.

An even more promising result was unexpectedly discovered by Stephen Lepore and his colleagues. They were conducting a writing study with young women college students who were coping with a recent romantic breakup. The idea of the study was to see if writing boosted the women's health. Although not intending to find anything beyond health improvements, Lepore found that the writing increased the odds that the women would get back together with their old partners.

Guided by Lepore's findings, Richard Slatcher ran a study of young college students who were in relationships and who texted each other daily. His idea was that he would get one member of the couple to either engage in expressive writing about their relationship or to write about superficial topics. Rich's team was curious about how expressive writing influenced the ways the couple texted. It turns out that expressive writing makes members of the couple more open and emotional with each other. But more striking, the study had a powerful effect on whether the couple stayed together.

A side note. Rich's study involved 86 couples, most of whom were college freshmen. As you might guess, first-year relationships are remarkably unstable. Three months after the study, about 77 percent of the couples in the expressive writing condition were still together, whereas only 52 percent of the controls were together. Who would have guessed? Pushing people to introspect about their relationship can make the relationship stronger. Will wonders never cease?

When Talking to Others Is Helpful versus Not Helpful

In 1976, Stanley Cobb, a researcher from the University of Michigan, published a groundbreaking article that said having a strong friendship network during times of stress can protect people's health. Across several large-scale studies, a strong social support network was found to protect people from illness and death following a wide range of tragedies. Hundreds, if not thousands, of studies have since supported and extended his early conclusions.

Over the years, we have begun to get a better sense of the power of social ties. A friendship network can buffer the effects of stress in a variety of ways. One of the most obvious is that friends can provide money, food, housing, or other tangible benefits if needed. They also can offer advice and an objective perspective to help people deal with problems in their lives. Hardly earth-shattering psychological news.

More interesting is that having a strong friendship network can help people maintain a stable view of their world and of themselves. One of the frightening aspects of traumas is that they cause us to question who we are. When a person unexpectedly loses her job due to layoffs, for example, she may try to understand it by saying to herself, "I deserved it; I am a bad person." Without friends, people are much more likely to blame themselves, as they have no other concrete information available to them. William Swann at the University of Texas at Austin has shown that, in times of crisis, people's self-esteem tends to be maintained by their friends. After a layoff, then, friends subtly bolster the person's world view by assuring her that she is, in fact, a good person.

Ironically, friends can also maintain some people's low self-esteem. People with low self-esteem have major difficulties dealing with success. If you have a negative view of yourself, you may become distressed if you receive a large raise or learn that others think you are a fascinating person. Interestingly, people with poor views of themselves who do not have a friendship circle have particularly severe health problems after success. With a friendship network, however, people with low self-esteem have fewer health problems following success because their "friends" assure them that they probably didn't deserve the success. In other words, a social network can keep us healthy by maintaining our self-views no matter what happens to us.

An amazing example of this can be seen with a student who had written a brilliant paper for one of our classes. The student had always had a very low opinion of himself and was genuinely surprised by the enthusiastic comments he received. A week later, he mentioned a letter from his father that said, in essence, "Anyone can write a psychology paper. Why did you make a B– in your accounting course?" The student's low self-esteem remained intact. He went on to become an accounting major.

In reality, most people have reasonably good feelings about themselves and also have access to social support. One benefit of social support is in providing an outlet for people to talk about their thoughts and feelings. In large surveys with corporate employees as well as college students, we find the same thing that other social support researchers have shown: the more friends you have, the healthier you are. However, this effect is due, almost exclusively, to the degree to which you have talked with your friends about any traumas that you have suffered.

But here is the kicker. If you have had a trauma that you have not talked about with anyone, the number of friends you have is unrelated to your health. Social support protects your health only if you use it wisely. That is, if you have suffered a major upheaval in your life, and you have supportive friends, talk to your friends about it. Merely having friends is not enough.

Choosing a Confidant

One reason that writing about upsetting experiences is a good coping strategy is that it is safe. If you use a journal to explore your thoughts and feelings, you can be completely honest with yourself. No one else will judge you, criticize you, or distort your perceptions of the world. Writing, however, has its drawbacks. It can be a slow and painful process. Many people find it difficult to express themselves on paper. Sometimes, people's perceptions of their own worlds can be distorted.

Ideally, we should be able to express all our most intimate thoughts to someone. But we can't. Even with our closest friends, there are usually some topics that we avoid because what we say might deeply hurt their feelings or make us look bad in their eyes. Is it possible to be totally honest with another person? Yes, sometimes. But there are several issues that must be considered before disclosing ourselves. In addition, there are important implications for a relationship when we let our guard down and honestly talk. (This also touches upon the issues of accepting personal vulnerability raised by Brené Brown that we noted earlier in Chapter 3.)

TRUST

Central to true self-disclosure is an overriding sense of trust. Jamie and his students examined the importance of trust in a project that they dubbed "the father confessor study." Students were asked to talk about their most traumatic experience for a few minutes while their physiological levels were monitored. Half of the students sat alone in a room and talked into a tape recorder. The other half spoke aloud to an anonymous psychology professor who sat on the other side of a curtain. Jamie was that professor. They never saw him, and he never saw them. They were told that he would just sit there and never respond to anything they said—all of which was true.

When alone, students let go and disclosed highly intimate parts of themselves. Indeed, their physiological measures, such as skin conductance levels, indicated that the highly disclosing students were not inhibiting what they said. The students talking to the anonymous father confessor, however, had physiological levels that were constantly elevated. They remained on guard the entire time. Afterward, they admitted that they didn't trust the person sitting on the other side of the curtain. One student, for example, noted that it was impossible that the father confessor was really a psychology professor because his shoes (which they could see) were shabby and cheap (!).

There is a certain irony in these findings. People readily opened up when talking into a tape recorder, even though they didn't know who would ever listen to the recording. When there was an anonymous person present, however, they became far more reticent in expressing their feelings and describing their experiences.

NONJUDGMENTAL RESPONSES FROM THE LISTENER

People are far more likely to disclose their feelings if they feel confident that others won't criticize what they say. Carl Rogers, the influential founder of client-centered therapy, maintained that the effectiveness of therapy hinged on a therapist who held the client in high regard no matter what was said. Even if a client had murdered his parents and robbed churches for a living, Rogers believed that it was critical for the therapist to accept the individual.

The logic of Rogers's approach is sound. If individuals honestly disclose their feelings about something, their feelings are real. To deny their feelings and perceptions is to deny the person. Several studies have found that when people are punished for disclosing their traumatic experiences, their psychological and physical health suffers.

THE SAFE BUT ANONYMOUS LISTENER

Several of the psychologists whom we know travel frequently. On planes, many avoid identifying themselves as psychologists because their fellow passengers often want to tell them everything about their lives. Both Josh and Jamie have heard innumerable shocking, heartbreaking, and fascinating stories. On one trip, a woman quietly confided her marital infidelity and unhappy marriage as her husband slept soundly next to her. Traveling psychologists are not the only ones to hear stories such as these. Studies suggest that bartenders, taxi drivers, prostitutes, and hairdressers serve as frequent listeners to people's confessions.

Why do people often tell their deepest thoughts and feelings to strangers but not to their spouses or friends? It's not that they trust the listeners or even that the listeners are nonjudgmental. Rather, according to classic work by the sociologist Georg Simmel, it is freedom from recrimination. If I want to talk to my airplane seatmate about my darkest secrets, I am safe with the knowledge that I will never see the person again. That knowledge is liberating. By definition, whatever I say will never affect any long-term relationship. Further, if the person is judgmental, it will have no ramifications.

THE PROFESSIONAL LISTENER

Before the growth of psychotherapy, people often disclosed their deepest secrets to their religious leaders, private physicians, or alternative healers such as palm or tea-leaf readers. In most cases, these professional listeners offered trust and confidentiality. Beginning in the 1950s, America and Europe witnessed a rapid expansion in the professionalization of listening. In 1960, for example, the annual number of newly minted clinical psychiatrists, psychologists, and counselors averaged under 500. By 1980, the number exceeded 4,000. By now, tens of thousands of new therapists appear on the scene each year.

At the same time that therapy was growing, other professions that had informally provided therapy declined in numbers or phased out the therapy role. In medicine, for example, there has been a drop in general or family practitioners. Church attendance has dropped. Even within many religions, the role of the minister or rabbi has changed. Many large congregations now employ a therapist to provide counseling. A fascinating expression of this change was seen in the Roman Catholic Church. Before the early 1970s, weekly private confessions were strongly encouraged. After the Second Vatican Council (Vatican II), however, the confession procedure became much more informal. The confession booth, or confessional, fast became relatively obsolete, with face-to-face meetings with the priest replacing it on an as-needed basis.

Psychotherapy offers a powerful setting for the disclosure of secrets, thoughts, and emotions. Therapists usually provide the essential ingredients of honest self-disclosure—trust, nonjudgmental feedback, and safety from recrimination—and distressed individuals also receive specific information on ways to cope with the source and symptoms of their stress. Therapy, like writing, can also help people feel better about themselves.

Professional listeners play a central role in our society. Large-scale studies indicate that psychotherapy in any form is effective in reducing physical health problems, depression, and an array of major and minor thought and behavior disorders. If you or a friend suffers from an intractable psychological problem, we *strongly* recommend psycho-therapy. Writing about your deepest thoughts and feelings should not be used as a substitute for therapy. Much like talking to a support-ive and trusted friend, writing is best viewed as a form of preventive maintenance.

IS TRANSFERENCE NECESSARY?

In developing psychoanalysis, Freud emphasized that therapy could be effective only if patients transferred their deepest or repressed emo-tions to the therapist. These basic emotions, which had usually been associated with a parent, were now the basis of a powerful attachment between the patient and the therapist. Often, when the transference of emotion occurs, the patient expresses deep love and/or hate toward the therapist. More recent forms of therapy still rely on the patient developing some type of emotional attachment to the therapist if ther-apy is to succeed.

In a sense, perhaps some degree of transference is necessary within a therapeutic relationship. As we have seen, however, thera-peutic gains can follow from writing or even from talking to a stranger on a plane—situations where transference is irrelevant. Freud and his followers may have confused therapy with a therapeutic relationship. When people begin therapy, for example, they know that they will be maintaining a close bond with the therapist for an extended amount of time. They must implicitly trust the therapist before they feel safe divulging their secrets.

The therapeutic dance occurs during the first few sessions of therapy, wherein the patients gauge their therapists' reactions, trust-worthiness, and competence. In any kind of ongoing relationship, the building of trust takes time. At first, patients indulge in a little stigma management. They divulge a little about themselves and carefully monitor the reaction of the therapist. Like the mating dances of birds or lovers, the patient and therapist go through a period of posturing before basic disclosure can occur. With writing or talking to strangers, the elements of disclosure are often immediately present.

FINAL CONSIDERATIONS IN CHOOSING A CONFIDANT

In our lives, we face a number of upsetting events that we want to discuss with someone. Divulging our deepest feelings can forge a powerful and lasting bond with others. Several experiments, for example, suggest that when one person discloses a secret to another, the other person often reciprocates. The interpersonal cycle of self-disclosure, according to social psychologists Irwin Altman and Dalmas Taylor, works much like the therapeutic dance between therapist and client. If neither person is rebuffed during the dance, the nature of disclosures becomes more intimate over time. Once the cycle is in place, the two people will have established a stable and trusting relationship that will provide an outlet for disclosure in case of future traumas.

But the dance can also pose psychological and social risks. People who unburden themselves and then are rejected by the listener can become depressed, hostile, and withdrawn. If you are currently living with a trauma and need to talk with someone, there are several safeguards that you should consider.

- *Self-disclosure will likely change the nature of your friendship.* Usually, revealing a deep secret will bring you and your friend closer. However, your friend may be threatened or hurt by what you say. If this happens, your relationship may be at risk. Telling your spouse about your desires for an extramarital affair, by way of example, may result in recrimination rather than understanding.

- *Hearing your traumas can be a trauma for the listener.* Oftentimes, the listener will need to discuss what you said with someone else. Secrets are contagious. According to research by Bernard Rimé at the University of Louvain in Belgium, the average secret told in confidence is spread to at least two other people. Gossip, although sometimes motivated by malice, can also reflect people's needs to discuss unsettling information with others.

- *Social blackmail exists.* Telling your dark secret can put the listener in a powerful position. The biblical story of Samson and Delilah serves as a nice illustration. Under God's orders, Samson was supposed to keep his secret that the source of his strength was his hair. In a weak moment, he confided his secret to his lover Delilah, who then sold the information to the Philistines. The upshot of Samson's poor judgment was that he lost his secret, his hair, and his strength.

- *The expectations of the listener can affect the content of the disclosure.* People can consciously or unconsciously change the ways they explain and interpret their deepest thoughts and feelings depending on their audience. The description of your feelings about a sexual trauma may variously emphasize guilt, powerlessness, or anger if your listener is a religious leader, psychologist, or the perpetrator. Ideally, your listener should allow you to explore all of your conflicting feelings about the event.

• *People's motivations for disclosing their secrets are not always pure.* Before disclosing an intimate secret to someone, ask yourself why you are choosing this particular person. It is common to see situations where people have truly hurt others by confiding. Although they claim to be acting in an honest and open way, their disclosures are clearly motivated by revenge. The tenor of the confession is often "You hurt me, so I am going to hurt you."

• *Telling and holding secrets can be a maladaptive substitute for taking action.* Many times, an upsetting experience can be corrected directly. As managers of research teams, both Jamie and Josh have witnessed cases where one person unintentionally hurt the feelings of another. The aggrieved individual often either stewed about the event or complained to others. In most of these cases, the entire incident could have been resolved if the aggrieved person simply expressed his or her feelings to the person who caused the problem in the first place. Most of us have observed similar processes in our professional and personal lives.

The Burden of Listening to Others' Traumas

A central theme of this chapter has centered on the distinction between confronting and being confronted by traumas. Psychologically confronting your own upheavals by talking about them can be healthy. Being confronted by someone else's trauma can be an emotional burden.

Indeed, listening to accounts of traumatic experiences may pose a health risk. Many years ago Jamie interviewed a large number of Holocaust survivors as part of a research project. He was not at all ready for the horrors that he would soon hear. About a week after interviewing his first two Holocaust survivors, he was devastated by a case of influenza. At the time, he was certain that his illness had nothing to do with stress—he had just been exposed to a flu virus, that's all. In looking back, there is good reason to believe that conducting the interviews, and the stress of hearing incredibly traumatic experiences, probably compromised his immune system, thereby making him more vulnerable to catching an infectious illness.

Over the last few decades, there have been dozens of studies demonstrating how listening to deeply troubling stories provokes significant stress responses. Whether watching people on television talk about terrible experiences or listening to others grappling with personal upheavals face to face, the process can make us nervous, angry, and helpless. In this light, you can begin to get a better appreciation of burnout.

Burnout was first examined in the late 1970s by Berkeley psychologist Christina Maslach. Individuals in many "people-work" occupations often report that, over time, they become emotionally exhausted and callous, and derive less satisfaction from their jobs. Professions with the highest rates of burnout include nursing, social work, and even sales and personnel positions. Each of these professions has traditionally had high turnover rates, greater than average absenteeism due to illness, and reports of job dissatisfaction.

Burnout, in many respects, is a problem of inhibition. One of the dangers of repeatedly being confronted by other people's traumas is that there is very little opportunity to talk about them. Particularly damaging, according to Maslach, is that burnout victims feel as though they have very little control over the lives of the people they talk with. This explains why physicians and therapists are less prone to burnout than similar groups, such as nurses, who have relatively less control. The more control the listener has in affecting the talker's life, the healthier the listener will be.

Listening to others' problems is an art form for which most of us have very little training. When psychologists and other people in the helping professions undergo training, they usually spend one or more years working under the close supervision of an experienced clinician. They discuss each of their cases in detail with their supervisor. This period of supervision serves as a training ground for keeping other people's secrets. Largely as a result of working in this area, both Jamie and Josh have listened to accounts of more traumas than most people will ever know about in a lifetime. It was hard at first not talking about them. Now, after years of conducting interviews and listening to stories, we can listen to nearly any kind of trauma at work and usually not think about it a single time when we get home.

Unfortunately, learning to suppress thoughts of other people's secret lives can take months or years. Assuming you don't want to spend the next few years in graduate school, how can you be a trustworthy listener when someone wants to tell you something intensely personal and upsetting? In posing this question to clinical psychologists, we have usually gotten two overlapping answers. The first is to write about it. (This may be a biased response, as the clinicians we have asked know about our research.) The second recommendation is to talk about it in veiled form to someone who doesn't know the person from whom you have heard the secret. You might consider calling a long-distance friend, for example. Remember, however, that talking it over with anyone always poses a risk because your behavior could be interpreted as a betrayal of trust.

The final strategy in listening to another's problems is knowing when to quit. When another person's trauma starts to become your trauma, your relationship with that person—as well as your own psychological and physical health—is at risk. You must honestly be able to admit to yourself and to the other person that you can no longer cope with his problem. Never be embarrassed to recommend a therapist or a support group. What may appear to be callous on the surface may also be far more helpful for your friend and you.

Personal Values Embedded within the Context

Try the following thought experiment. Imagine that we asked you to write down your very deepest thoughts and feelings concerning your personal feelings of sexuality and love.

• *Scenario 1*. Imagine that you will keep your writing and no one will ever see what you have written. Before we change scenes, seriously think to yourself how you would go about writing on this particular topic. What secret issues and hidden desires would you bring up?

• *Scenario 2*. Imagine this time that we will be giving your writing sample to your parents and will be asking them to evaluate what you have written on sexuality and love. For some people, the writing style for this scenario would be relatively similar to that for the first one. Most, however, would subtly—or dramatically—change the content and style of what they had written.

• *Scenarios 3, 4, etc.* Imagine the same writing assignment, but this time your essay, which, of course, would have your name on it, would be read by your boss. Or your minister or rabbi. Or maybe the sophomore class at the local high school. Or even a convention of psychologists who would judge your mental health.

You get the idea. We can all honestly divulge our deepest thoughts and feelings to different audiences. However, we change our definition of "deepest" depending on the audience. We also subtly alter our interpretations of identical events from setting to setting.

There are some obvious reasons that people's stories change depending on the audience. If individuals think that the intended audience would disapprove or could, in some way, punish them, they will almost have to reconstruct their stories. Similarly, if the intended audience is personally or professionally important, people will bend their essays to make them look as good as possible. But the seeking of rewards and the avoidance of punishment is only one type of motivation that guides how we write and talk about our personal experiences.

Within any given social situation, there are a number of unspoken but tacitly agreed-upon values. When you enter a religious establishment, for example, no one needs to give you a written list of approved behaviors. Even if you have never been in that particular house of worship, you instantly know that you shouldn't smoke, drink alcohol, laugh boisterously, and so forth. Similarly, if you go to meet with a bank officer in an attempt to get a loan, there are some topics that you avoid. The overarching values in the religious establishment may be *respect* and *tradition*. In the bank foyer, the tacit values might be *frugality* and *fiscal responsibility*.

The importance of settings is that they can engage an entire set of implicit values. These values are the ones by which you may measure yourself at that particular time. For example, if a college professor versus a bank officer asked you to evaluate your own personality, your thinking about your own intelligence would flow more naturally in front of the professor and your ideas about money management skills would tend to surface in front of the bank officer. The setting or the context, then, is laden with implicit values that can shape our disclosures.

Testing Out the Influence of Implicit Values

Try writing about your deepest thoughts and feelings about yourself for 2 minutes. You can keep anything you write and never show it to a soul. But imagine first that the person asking you to write is a psychologist. Then write as if the person requesting the writing is a religious leader. The mere identity of the person making the request will alter the implicit values that are prominent in your own mind. Consequently, the way you write will likely change even though the person giving the instructions will never see your writing sample.

The implicit values for the psychologist might be for you to explore your own thoughts from a psychology perspective—whatever that might be. At the back of your mind, for example, you might ask yourself, "Am I sane? Do I get along with people well? Did I have a normal childhood?" These can be central questions that, when answered, give us a better understanding of ourselves.

The implicit values associated with the religious leader may be equally central to our being but may be quite different from those linked to the psychologist. If the religious person asked you to explore your own thoughts and feelings, the implicit values of the situation might prompt you to ask yourself, "Am I a good person? Do I treat others honestly and fairly? Was I a good child for my parents?" Any self-reflective essay, then, would elicit answers to questions that were implicitly aroused by the religious context.

You can see, then, how our efforts to explain traumas will be strongly influenced by invoking different implicit values. As a thought exercise, assume, for example, that you have been the victim of a serious home invasion and violent assault—and are now trying to grapple with this highly threatening and potentially overwhelmingly traumatic experience. Indeed, whether you are a psychologist, minister, or Maoist-inspired communist, you will have no ready understanding of such a trauma. In all likelihood, you will obsess about it, dream about it, develop irrational fears about it, and probably suffer from several physical illnesses in the year after the trauma.

Now imagine being asked to write anonymously about your traumatic experience within the context of either implicit psychological, religious, or political values. From the psychological perspective, many of the issues you would write about would explore why you currently felt the way you did. Using the religious value system, you might address acceptance of hardships as in the Book of Job. From a political point of view, you might explain your and the perpetrator's behaviors as reflecting the political or economic system. No matter what value system you adopted, however, you would probably benefit from the writing experience. By translating the event into language, you would now have a better understanding of the event and of yourself.

The irony of writing from any of the three perspectives is that your understanding of the experience will be completely different depending on the context in which you write. There would also be another important change in your own mind after writing: You would adhere to the implicit value system to a far greater extent than before your writing.

When we write or talk about a trauma, we tend to use whatever implicit and explicit values are available to help us try to understand it. If, for example, we were asked to confide to a respected pastor in the community, we very likely would try to explain our trauma by way of implicit religious values. The mere act of doing this would define the trauma in semireligious terms. The implicit values of religion, in this example, would be used to define a centrally important psychological event in our life—the trauma. If this implicit value *can* explain the trauma, we will be likely to invoke the same value system in the future to explain other traumas. The original implicit values aroused by our confiding in a pastor will have now become a central way in which we define ourselves.

Confession in context, then, becomes a very powerful psychological force. When people disclose deeply personal experiences within a given context, they will be likely to define their personalities, their very selves, in line with the values of the context. Confession is not necessarily dangerous in and of itself. It does have the potential for danger when people start to understand and define themselves using only the implicit values surrounding the context of their disclosures. This may be part of why anonymous writing can be so powerful—because it allows the writer/discloser to develop his or her own understanding of the traumatic event independent of any particular value system (recognizing, of course, that people bring their own values to bear). Conversely, when confessing or disclosing in a context, it may be useful to be aware of any constraints this may evoke—and to try not to censor yourself based on this context, allowing yourself a fuller and freer processing of the event.

CHAPTER 9

How Does Writing Help Us Secure a Healthier and Happier Future?

We hope you are persuaded that brief writing or talking about powerful emotional experiences or events can change people's physical and mental health over the subsequent weeks and months. Hundreds of studies in countries all over the world have now demonstrated the power of translating emotional upheavals into words. We now return to a difficult and important question: How can this possibly work? Why does writing produce such beneficial effects? Although we have addressed components of this in passing, this issue deserves more detailed attention.

Recall that keeping secrets appears to require considerable physiological work. Originally, many researchers felt that writing reduced the work of inhibition. That is, if holding in secrets was physiologically tiring, releasing them through expressive writing should therefore help by removing this burden. Virtually no studies directly supported this idea. When people were asked why writing had helped them, many spontaneously said that they came to a new understanding of the emotional events themselves. Problems that had seemed overwhelming became simpler and more manageable after seeing them on paper. Writing helped to resolve problems. Once the issues were resolved, there was no need to think about them anymore.

The Need for Completion and the Search for Meaning

That we remember, think about, and dream of unresolved issues has been a central feature of psychological study for many decades. In 1927, Bluma Zeigarnik and her mentor Kurt Lewin found that people had a far better memory for interrupted tasks than completed ones. For example, if you are interrupted just before the end of an exciting movie, you will remember the movie more vividly and for a longer time than if you saw the movie's resolution. People have a basic need for completing and resolving tasks. The tasks may be as trivial as buttoning all of your buttons in the morning or as profound as resolving the major conflicts you have with your parents or children.

We all tend to think and dream about unresolved matters or about tasks that are not quite completed. In the last hour, for example, you may have had fleeting thoughts about your mother's health, what you will have for dinner, the battery problem you are having on your phone, whether you should sign up for foreign language lessons, and dozens of other minor and major issues. Once each of these issues is resolved, you will cease thinking about it. You will stop thinking about your mother's health once she is well and the battery in your phone once it is replaced. When your family or friends get together over the soon-to-be-decided dinner, you will each talk about what happened today. Many, perhaps most, of the issues that will be brought up will be those that are not yet fully resolved or understood. Finally, the dreams that you have tonight will probably reflect certain unresolved fears, urges, or thoughts that you are currently living with.

Major tasks or goals in our lives are difficult to resolve or complete. Consider what researchers find to be some of the more common life tasks that we set for ourselves: to love and to be loved; to make the world a better place; to raise healthy and happy children; to succeed professionally and financially; to be honest with ourselves and others. As if these tasks weren't difficult enough to accomplish, imagine the problems we face when confronted with an overwhelming trauma. Divorce, death of a loved one, financial ruin, public humiliation, or some other upheaval can disrupt an entire series of life tasks. If our marriage is falling apart, for example, we have to deal with our life goals of being permanently married, being loved, raising happy children, succeeding financially, and so forth. Traumas, according to this approach, represent interruptions of life tasks.

If people naturally seek completion of disrupted tasks, the changes that occur following an unexpected trauma become far more understandable. Among people in the midst of a divorce, it makes good sense that they would ruminate, talk, and dream about the many aspects of their lives touched by the breakup of their relationship. Thoughts and dreams have long been considered symbolic ways of completing unresolved life tasks. One function of dreams, Freud claimed, was wish fulfillment. More recent thinkers have suggested that dreams can help us work through uncompleted life tasks.

But thoughts and dreams do more than attain completion of a disrupted task. If our closest friend is killed by a drunk driver, we also have to accept that the event happened and that our lives will inexorably be different than we had planned. Our thoughts wander from "if only I had done this or if my friend had done that" to asking why this happened. In other words, we seek to understand why the event occurred. More broadly, we try to find meaning to the event and, perhaps, life itself.

A motivation closely akin to the need for completion is the basic need to understand the world around us. This need for understanding and meaning is probably central to most vertebrates. A mouse that narrowly escapes the jaws of the neighborhood cat needs to know what factors predict the presence of the cat and how to avoid the cat in the future. A toddler who is yelled at for sticking her finger in the direction of an electrical outlet seeks to understand the meaning of the yell. As our mental apparatus becomes more sophisticated, our search for the meaning of events becomes more intensive. We go to great lengths to understand such things as why we got that parking ticket or why our boss turned down our entirely reasonable request for a raise.

Making Sense of Our World

In our culture—perhaps all cultures—the key to understanding is learning what causes what. Usually, if we can isolate the cause of something that we couldn't figure out up to then, we are satisfied. We have attained a form of psychic completion. For example, if the new nail clippers we ordered online have not arrived by the delivery date, we have to ask ourselves why. What could explain this relatively minor event? Possible explanations that might go through our minds are that the address on the package was wrong; it was delivered and some passerby stole it; it wasn't delivered due to the delivery person's negligence; maybe we didn't really order the nail clippers; maybe this isn't our house. Once we can isolate any of these possibilities as the cause, we can take corrective action. Once we understand the problem and have received our nail clippers, we can put the entire episode behind us without giving it another thought.

We are driven to complete tasks and to understand our worlds. These motives serve us well until we are faced with massive, overwhelming traumatic experiences. This is especially true for unpredictable events that can never be truly explained. Think back to the example of a close friend killed by a drunk driver. By definition, you can never complete your relationship with your friend by saying goodbye. Further, it is difficult if not impossible to find any meaning in the event. Nevertheless, our brains are constructed and/or our minds are trained to move toward completion and to find meaning.

Some religions offer answers to meaningless tragedies: "God has a plan" or "I will see my friend when I eventually die." Others take a more detached perspective by noting that death is merely an evolution of the life force. Several researchers have found that people who can turn to their personal religious beliefs—no matter what the actual religion may be—fare better in the face of certain traumas than those who are not religious.

The issue goes far beyond religion, however. We are often so intent on finding meaning in an event that we become irrational. Several intriguing experiments have demonstrated that if we see someone who is physically abused for no reason, we tend to come up with a reason. A ready explanation is to blame the victim, which is most likely to occur among people who believe that the world is fundamentally just and fair. The more you think the world is just, the more invested you are in rationalizing unfair occurrences to others. Such reasoning is able to maintain people's beliefs that we live in a just world.

Among those who can easily explain all bad things, whether through strongly held religious beliefs or more paranoid blame-the-victim belief systems, feelings of anxiety are not a problem. The majority of people in Western society, however, have drifted away from simple cause–effect explanations for tragedies and traumas. With the awareness that the world is ambiguous and unpredictable comes the anxiety of not attaining closure and not understanding many events.

And therein lies the problem. We naturally search for meaning and completion to events that we know at some level don't have meaning and can never be resolved. We are too smart for our own good but can't admit it. In fact, studies among women who were incest victims as children reveal that the search for meaning can in some cases be both futile and unhealthy. Roxane Silver, for example, cites evidence to suggest that the 50 percent of former incest victims who continue to search for meaning report never making any sense of it. As two incest victims wrote:

"I always ask myself why, over and over, but there is no answer."

"It is useful to have the past in mind, but not always. It can stimulate thought but can also keep one from really listening and learning in the present."

Understanding the Unfathomable

Work with incest, rape, and other trauma victims by Ronnie Janoff-Bulman of the University of Massachusetts at Amherst suggested that it is usually easy to answer a question like "Why did the sexual trauma occur?" It is much harder to answer "Why did it happen to me?" According to Janoff-Bulman, victims of traumas may often answer these questions by blaming themselves, saying, in essence, "I deserved it." Again, you can see how this happens. People have a desperate need to understand an event that may not have any real meaning. After thinking about various explanations, people may opt for the simple explanation that they brought it on themselves. Although a self-blaming explanation may be inaccurate and personally devastating, at least it makes the person's world more understandable.

The mind torments itself with thoughts about unresolved and confusing issues. Childhood sexual abuse survivors report extremely high rates of self-blame and feelings of shame. Those who are able to talk with others tend to fare much better than those who keep the experiences to themselves. Talking, like expressive writing, may help the survivors find meaning or, at the very least, help them reach some kind of self-understanding.

Some of the evidence about the role of writing in helping individuals resolve upsetting experiences comes from the participants in early experiments. Months after people had written about traumas, over 70 percent reported that writing helped them understand both the event and themselves better. A typical volunteer in the first writing experiment, for example, responded to a questionnaire mailed to her five months after the study:

> *I had to think and resolve past experiences. . . . One result of the experiment is peace of mind, and a method to relieve emotional experiences. To have to write emotions and feelings helped me understand how I felt and why.*

Words such as *realize, understand, resolve,* and *work through* appear in approximately half of the open-ended responses that were received to questions about the general value of the writing experiments. Intuitively, people see writing as a method by which to understand and resolve personal upheavals. Their intuitions are probably accurate. What they don't tell us is how writing accomplishes these cognitive changes.

The secret may lie in how we naturally think about things. If we analyze our day on a minute-by-minute basis, we are able to resolve, understand, or perhaps ignore almost everything that confronts us: why there is a squeak in the chair; why the coffee is especially bitter; why the electricity bill is so high. Our minds are ideally suited to simple and even moderately complex problems. But traumas are a different matter. The events themselves may be so intricate that attaining any understanding may be nearly impossible, yet their effects cannot be ignored.

Losing Your Job: Brian's Story

A striking example of the confusion faced by people when they suddenly are thrust into a psychic maelstrom can be seen in the case of a man laid off by an oil company for which he had worked for 21 years. Brian, a 43-year-old geologist who had volunteered for a writing study, wrote about his predicament:

> *I have always loved my job, this company, and the people I work with. All our friends are with the company. Now, after two decades I receive a notice that falling oil prices have forced them to do away with my entire office. We will have to move into a cheaper house, maybe to a new town. I even have*

to think about switching occupations. . . . It is so demeaning. Other people think I am a loser. I feel like it sometimes, too.

In the last month, my world has turned upside down. My identity, my friends, my moods, my time. As soon as I start thinking about one change in my life, some other aspect occurs to me. It is impossible to keep my attention on much of anything for more than a few minutes. Anger, depression, bitterness. . . . Sometimes brief bursts of optimism. I have never had so many moods in one day. Why did this happen?

The enormity of losing his job touched virtually every aspect of Brian's life. No matter how intelligent Brian may have been, it is unlikely that he could have sorted out all of the issues while moping around his house or during the many hours he spent watching television.

In Brian's case, writing appeared to help because it forced some degree of structure and organization of his thoughts. When he wrote, his thinking process was forced to slow down. Before writing, he would have one thought very rapidly followed by another and another; their totality was too much to deal with: it was overwhelming. No thought or emotion was ever resolved. When he began writing, however, he was able to follow an idea to its logical conclusion. Indeed, as his writing progressed day by day, he began to focus on specific topics in an orderly manner. By the third day of his writing he disclosed his anxieties about being unemployed and not making money; another session was devoted to the added tension that he was experiencing with his wife; soon he was focusing on his social and professional skills in order to assess his possibilities in alternative careers.

Another common phenomenon that occurs when people write about the same trauma repeatedly is a gradual change in perspective. Over time, individuals who are writing about a specific event tend to become more and more detached. They are able to stand back and consider the complex causes of the event and their own mixed emotions. Perhaps by addressing the trauma multiple times, writing makes people's emotional responses become less extreme. In other words, repeatedly confronting an upsetting experience allows for a less emotionally laden assessment of its meaning and impact; it appears to offer a bit more distance and perspective.

Other research finds that it is important that people be able to freely express their emotions, particularly if doing so to others. Actively holding back feelings, whether because one perceives or actually experiences others responding negatively, can be stressful. A large number of studies have shown that these perceived or actual restrictions on one's ability to disclose emotions and feelings, also called social constraints, are indeed detrimental to one's physical and psychological health (you may recall this issue from elsewhere in the book, notably Chapter 8). In addition, admitting our emotions to ourselves and others serves an important communicative function. If I am angry because of an underhanded comment by a friend, for example, it is important that I recognize my feelings so that I can direct my actions in an acceptable way. I can also let my friend know how I feel so that she can gauge the intended impact of the comment on me.

Many therapists today believe that it is valuable for individuals to achieve some understanding of the causes and consequences of the traumatic experiences that affect them. By talking or otherwise disclosing about upsetting events, people achieve insight into the events and learn more about themselves. With this knowledge, it is thought, people can better put the traumas behind them by changing thoughts, feelings, and/or behaviors that may be arising from difficulty with the traumatic experience. For instance, Jennifer Graham and her colleagues at Pennsylvania State University asked chronic pain patients to disclose their experiences by writing a letter about something they were angry about. Those who were seen to be engaging in more "meaning making" in these letter disclosures (understanding the conditions and reasons that led to their anger) had lower rates of depression two months later.

But what might promote this process of meaning making? Ethan Kross and Ozlem Adyuk have done fascinating work exploring factors that may facilitate meaning making when thinking about negative experiences. In particular, they have found that the perspective (or point of view) one takes is important in determining more helpful, or adaptive, thinking versus unhelpful rumination, worry, and distress. For example, taking a third-party perspective (how someone else would see the situation) seems to provide some emotional distance, and facilitates the processing of negative experiences and leads to enhanced understanding and meaning. In addition, the benefits of this kind of perspective taking appear to emerge when thinking (and presumably writing) about the causes and consequences of the events, but less so if focusing only on the negative feelings associated with the event. In fact, their work suggests focusing solely on negative emotions may even be harmful in some circumstances.

Looking for the Positive: Benefit Finding

Finding meaning in a complex event is not an easy task. In fact, there are several ways one can determine meaning. One strategy is to try to reinterpret upsetting experiences. Rather than just focus on the hardship, pain, and misery of a miserable experience, there is some evidence that looking at the positive sides of it may have merit. It is an interesting idea. Let's be honest, most truly wonderful experiences have some downsides. It follows that most bad experiences have some good sides. Can people's health improve if they look for the benefits in misfortune?

There is some evidence to support such an idea. In one study, university students were asked to write about the loss of a loved one. Some of the students were randomly assigned to try to find meaning in the loss; the remaining students were asked to try to look on the bright side of the loss—a concept called benefit finding. The study found relatively powerful benefits for emotional disclosure of any kind—students showed not only better physical health, but also lower rates of prolonged grief, depressive symptoms, and posttraumatic stress symptoms. Most important, these benefits were even a bit stronger in the benefit-finding condition than for those asked to find meaning in the loss.

Laura King from the University of Missouri, a particularly influential figure in the study of personality, has proposed that people can find value by casting emotional upheavals into their broader conceptions of who they would like to be. In an important study, she asked individuals to disclose through writing their thoughts and feelings about their "best possible future self":

> "Think about yourself in the future. Imagine that everything has gone as well as it possibly could. Think of this as the realization of all your life dreams. Now, write about what you imagined."

Individuals writing in response to the prompt above showed reductions in physician visits over the following months. Notably, these benefits were more pronounced in this study than those experienced by respondents asked to just write about a trauma they had experienced (i.e., the more typical expressive writing instructions).

A number of researchers since have continued to explore writing methods that broadly fall under the umbrella of self-regulation. The idea is that expressive writing may enhance one's ability to pursue goals in more effective ways. With the right instructions, writing has the ability to boost people's feelings of self-efficacy, mastery of emotion, and accomplishment with the net effect of improving health and well-being. For instance, Linda Cameron and Gregory Nicholls conducted a research study that asked respondents to disclose a problem and explore possible solutions. Those asked to do so benefit similarly to those asked to disclose their thoughts and feelings more directly.

Engaging in positive psychological processes, whether benefit finding or problem solving, while expressing emotions appears to be a good way of coping with stress. Can people attain insight through disclosing per se? Many directive therapists, who have been strongly influenced by Freud and his followers, believe that talking helps to achieve insight in no small part due to the comments of the therapist. That is, tell them your problems and they will help you figure out what is really going on. Once the underlying emotionally charged difficulties have been isolated, they will do what they can to clear them up. Other more nondirective therapies, such as Carl Rogers's client-centered therapy, suggest that by your telling the therapist what is bothering you, you will be able to figure out your own problems and solutions. The therapist, in this case, will be a sounding board who is accepting and trustworthy no matter what you say.

A number of clinical techniques, although quite different in their theoretical underpinnings and how they approach therapy, have been found to be effective in the treatment of most psychological disorders. Attaining insight into our own thoughts and feelings must be valuable. After all, if I know why I feel depressed in one kind of situation or nauseated in another, I can take steps to master or avoid those situations. Further, I can try to change myself so I won't react the way I do or, if I cannot change, my reactions will at least be predictable.

The Role of Translating Experiences into Language

Many first-time teachers have had the experience of becoming a bit dense when they begin explaining things to their students. A seasoned teacher explains the phenomenon:

The public unveiling of my ignorance in my role as teacher occurred during my second lecture where I planned to talk about how psychologists measure relationships among two variables using a statistic called a correlation coefficient. I had used, computed, and interpreted correlations for years and assumed that I would simply explain how these statistics worked.

I stood in front of the class and began to describe what a correlation was. Within a minute or two, I realized my explanation made absolutely no sense. I tried another tack—again, what I was saying was absurd. By my third attempt, students began asking very reasonable questions that I could only answer with mumbles. I remember looking out at the students as I stammered incoherently and thinking to myself, "My God, I honestly don't understand correlations."

If you can't explain something to someone else, you probably don't understand it yourself. If it can be true for someone who used correlation coefficients most days in his research, it can also be true for personal experiences. Translating a phenomenon, particularly a complex one, into clear language fundamentally alters the way it is represented and understood in our minds.

The failure or inability to translate traumatic experiences into language has been implicated as one possible cause of PTSD. Whereas the failure to translate powerful emotions into language appears to be psychologically unhealthy, linking our emotional memories to language is often beneficial. One treatment for individuals suffering from PTSD is the use of active talk therapies wherein sufferers are asked to relive and talk about their emotional upheavals.

The central idea is that when we convert an image in our minds into words, it fundamentally alters the way the image is stored. Jonathan Schooler, now at the University of California at Santa Barbara, did an ingenious experiment to demonstrate this. Students in an experiment were shown pictures of people's faces and told to remember them as best they could. People were asked to describe some of the pictures but not others. In other words, some of the pictures were translated into language whereas others were not.

Schooler discovered that the students were less likely to remember the pictures that were described in words than the others. Apparently, once an image is translated into language, it becomes degraded and altered in memory, making it harder to recall what the actual image was like. Talking about the image involves additional, different parts of the brain than when one is focusing on the image alone. As a result, the face, not unlike emotional events that are not discussed, may well be stored in a nonlanguage form. It follows that translating abstract thoughts and emotions associated with a traumatic event into written words with a linguistic structure may allow for the traumatic event to be better understood and integrated into one's understanding of "self" and the world. As a result, when the trauma is recalled, the experiences are more linguistic and narrative in nature; this helps to reduce the emotional intensity and impact of the experiences.

Language can be thought of as a tool that simplifies experience. Think of a time that you have told the same story to different people over and over again. Right after Jamie's wife, Ruth, had their first baby, they excitedly talked about the birth in detail with their relatives and friends. It was such an emotional and unique event in their lives that they relished telling about their childbirth adventure. One thing they both noticed was that the account of the event subtly changed over time. Initially, it was a jumble of sights, sounds, emotions, and thoughts—both in their minds and in the ways they talked about it. Later, the experience became more of a story, with a clear beginning and end. Even the story itself changed, becoming shorter and more concise. The act of repeatedly telling about their experience resulted in both an organization to the event and a summarizing of it.

A similar phenomenon occurs in experiments when people write about the same trauma several days in a row. The description of the event is gradually shortened and summarized. Irrelevant issues and tangential impressions are dropped; central features of the traumas are highlighted and analyzed. The experimental volunteers have created a mental summary of their experience that often is psychologically less daunting to deal with. One woman, after writing about being raped by a casual acquaintance, explained:

I haven't been able to talk about the rape in detail to anyone. In the last three months, it has dominated my being. I've had fears and problems with other people that I've never had before. Being in this [writing experiment] has made a difference. Somehow, just writing about what happened has made it all less overwhelming. I won't ever forget what happened but I see more clearly that it was an isolated event in my life.

Summarizing and Sharing Memory to Reduce Stress

Nearly any type of an event is less overwhelming and easier to think about once it is summarized in some way. Many times, when we write something down, we don't have to think about it any longer. You may have noticed this when you are preparing to go on a vacation. There's packing, stopping the mail, getting the car checked, and on and on. In the middle of meetings or talking to someone on the phone, overlooked chores come to mind. "Oh, I can't forget to pack the fishing rod" or "get someone to water the plants." As much as you try to avoid it, you probably break down and start making lengthy lists of last-minute tasks to perform. Before list making, you have to actively juggle the tasks in your mind. Once you start the lists, however, your mind becomes freer and you probably feel a little less distressed. You have, in essence, transferred your mental notes from your head onto a piece of paper.

Several researchers have discussed how memory and thought processes can be viewed as external to our brains. Dan Wegner provided fascinating examples of how partners in a marriage gradually become repositories of each other's thoughts and memories. One spouse may remember restaurants; the other may keep track of movies. One spouse never has to think about finances, for example, because all financial thoughts are housed in the other spouse's brain.

As with list making or marriage, we can also construe the act of writing about a trauma as a method of externalizing a traumatic experience. Once it has been written down or told to another, the memory and value of it have been preserved. There is now less of a reason to rehearse the event actively. In the computer world, this is analogous to transferring data from one computer system to another; it removes the file(s) and frees up space on the original computer, and relocates the information to the second computer. Both Jamie and Josh found in their early writing studies that at least one participant typically asked to keep his or her essays. These participants report that what they have written is a part of themselves and that they want to be able to refer back to their thoughts and feelings in the future. They have downloaded their traumas but don't want their memories destroyed—in this metaphor, they want the source files preserved on their own computer.

The Drive toward Self-Expression

Individuals have been known to produce major literary works while under great conflict. Eugene O'Neill's *Long Day's Journey into Night*, Sylvia Plath's *The Bell Jar*, Cheryl Strayed's *Wild*, and many other masterpieces express the fundamental psychological fears and traumas of the authors. A parallel phenomenon occurs within the visual arts, music composition, and dance. The stark photography of Diane Arbus, the twisted visions of van Gogh, the conflicted musical themes of Gustav Mahler or Kurt Cobain, or the haunting choreography of Alvin Ailey or Bob Fosse attests to the expression of conflicts across a variety of media.

Is there a basic human need to express ourselves? One highly respected scholar, Abraham Maslow, suggested that if our most basic needs—such as food, sex, and security—are satisfied, people exhibit a strong drive toward self-expression. When this drive is blocked, tension will result. One reason that writing about traumas may be physically healthy is that writing itself is a fundamental form of self-expression.

Writing, of course, is only one of many forms of self-expression. Looking back to our previous experiments, would people have shown similar improvements in physical health if they had been asked to draw, sing, or dance about their most upsetting experiences? This has been an important question in the creative and expressive arts.

Expression through Dancing and Drawing

In a striking article published in the *American Journal of Public Health* in 2010, Heather Stuckey and Jeremy Nobel summarized dozens of studies that explored whether singing, dancing, drawing, painting, acting, or writing stories or poetry could improve health. Most of the studies were impressionistic or case studies, but a small number were scientifically sound. As the authors pointed out, the findings were promising but not conclusive (a conclusion echoed by similar reviews conducted since). More than anything, this review highlighted the need for rigorous research with carefully assessed biological or behavioral outcomes to be conducted.

One study is particularly relevant—one that was conducted by

Anne Krantz, a dance therapist in San Francisco. The study itself was quite simple. Sixty-four students participated in a study on "bodily movement." They were randomly assigned either to express a traumatic experience using bodily movement, to express an experience using movement and then write about it for 10 additional minutes, or to exercise in a prescribed manner (much like in an exercise class). Each of these was done every day for three consecutive days, for at least 10 minutes each session. Although the people in the two expressive movement groups were unsupervised and "danced" without music, they reported that they enjoyed the movement more than those who performed the movement routines. Whereas the people in the two movement expression groups reported that they felt happier and healthier in the months after the study, only the movement group that also wrote evidenced improvements in physical health and grade-point average. The mere expression of a trauma was not sufficient. Health gains appeared to require translating experiences into some narrative or language.

Emotional disclosure through drawing may also be helpful. Jennifer Drake at Brooklyn College has shown that expressive drawing can be used to promote positive emotion regulation in children. Among people who feel at ease drawing, informal studies in our labs find reductions in physiological levels while dealing with emotional topics. Some people have further noted that they paint or draw when they are depressed. Again, for most, the experience seems to be more emotional than cognitive. As one artist friend explained:

> If I am bummed out, I'll pick up my pad and start to sketch. When I do it, I stop thinking and just draw. Sometimes I'm not even aware of what I am drawing until I have been going for a few minutes. Yes, it can be really cathartic and emotionally draining. It can also be kind of a distraction as well. Maybe it's more of a meditative state.

It is not coincidental that there are a variety of therapies that use self-expressive techniques unrelated to writing. As noted, dance therapy, art therapy, and music therapy have gained widespread popularity and are used with children and adults. There is good reason to believe that these alternative approaches are beneficial. Their effectiveness, however, is not merely in fulfilling self-expressive needs.

Dance, art, and music therapies can be powerful in getting individuals to experience emotions related to relevant upheavals in their lives. Expressive movement, drawing, or singing can undoubtedly strip away inhibitions and other defenses. In this state, people are more emotionally aware but not necessarily closer to an understanding of their thoughts and feelings. Indeed, most dance, art, and music therapists go far beyond encouraging self-expression. During or after dancing, drawing, or singing, clients are strongly encouraged to talk about their emotional experiences. In other words, non-language-based therapies often rely heavily on language once the clients' inhibitions are lifted.

Words Matter

Most of the evidence supporting the therapeutic value of writing points to the importance of translating emotional experiences into language. Over the years, we and many others have hypothesized that understanding the causes of an upsetting event, together with some degree of self-reflection or insight, is necessary to health improvement. These are very reasonable hypotheses. Unfortunately, a reasonable hypothesis isn't worth much without solid evidence.

In theory, it should be possible to see how writing brings about psychological change by tracking people's writing samples. Surely, there must be clues in the ways people write that could identify healthy writing styles. Some early work involved multiple experts reading expressive writing essays to determine dimensions of language that reflected the psychological states of the authors. No luck. It turns out to be almost impossible for anyone to identify healthy or unhealthy writing. There are just too many dimensions of language.

A few years after the first expressive writing papers had been published, a revolution in computer technology and Internet access to language samples was under way. It was now possible to build simple computer programs that could go into any typed essay, analyze a very large array of language dimensions, and begin sorting out healthy from unhealthy writing. Working with one of his graduate students, Martha Francis, Jamie helped develop a computer program called Linguistic Inquiry and Word Count, or LIWC.

Without going too much into the details, the LIWC program could analyze any essay, book, newspaper article, or any (transcribed) verbal utterance almost immediately. The beauty of LIWC was that it computed the percentage of words in a given file that reflected various positive and negative emotions as well as general thinking styles. In fact, LIWC analyzed language along more than seventy different dimensions.

More on Language

www.secretlifeofpronouns.com

With the help of LIWC, we analyzed all of the written essays from six earlier writing studies to see if we could predict improved health by isolating the word categories people used. Three linguistic factors emerged that were related to better subsequent health:

- Higher rates of positive emotion words (including words such as *happy*, *love*, *good*, and *laugh*)
- A moderate number of negative emotion words (e.g., *angry*, *hurt*, and *ugly*)
- An increasing use of cognitive or thinking words over the course of writing

In fact, the increasing use of cognitive words showed the strongest relationship to later improvements in physical health. Cognitive words tapped causal thinking (e.g., words such as *cause*, *effect*, *reason*) and insight or self-reflection (e.g., *understand*, *realize*, *know*). Interestingly, it wasn't the actual level of word use for these categories that was important. Rather, those people who showed improvements in health went from using fewer cognitive words on the first day of writing to using more cognitive words on the last day of writing.

The cognitive word effects were in line with our expectations that writing was helping people make sense of their experiences. It reflected the fact that people were working to put a story or narrative together.

Another language finding was discovered a few years later. By analyzing people's use of pronouns (words such as *I*, *we*, *you*, *she*, *they*), it was possible to determine where their attention was focused. It was discovered that people whose health improved the most tended to change their perspective from one writing session to the next. So, for example, a writer who talked about his or her feelings on the first day of writing and then focused on other people on the second day would be more likely to show health improvements than someone who had the same perspective every day of writing.

Using our computer analyses as a guide, we realized that the people who benefited from writing were naturally constructing stories on their own, without explicit directions to do so. On the first day of their writing, they would often tell about a traumatic episode by simply describing an experience, often out of sequence and disorganized. But day by day as they continued to write, the episode would take on shape as a coherent story with a clear beginning, middle, and end. Ironically, participants who started the study with a clear, coherent, and well-organized story rarely evidenced any health improvements.

What these patterns of effects were suggesting was that people who benefit from writing change in the ways they write over the course of the expressive writing sessions. They are exhibiting a certain kind of cognitive growth. They are testing and developing a new story to explain their emotional upheavals. People who write the same way every day are more likely in a rut—they are telling the same story over and over without changing it.

As a side note, the LIWC program has since developed into a very powerful tool and is used in a variety of ways within psychology, medicine, business, and other disciplines. Language use has been found to reflect personality, the quality of social relationships, honesty, depression, and other states and traits.

The Role of Narrative

Our hypotheses are no longer just interesting speculation. People who benefit most from translating their experiences into language tend to write in a particular way. Just as we are drawn to good stories in literature or the movies, we need to construct coherent and meaningful stories for ourselves. Good narratives or stories, then, organize the seemingly infinite facets of overwhelming events. Once organized, the events are often smaller and easier to deal with. Particularly important is that writing moves us to a resolution. Even if there is no meaning to an event, it becomes psychologically complete. In short, there is no more reason to continue to ruminate about it.

At the same time that Jamie was delving into the nature of language, Josh was attempting to understand how essays on traumatic topics were organized. His thinking was similar, based on the idea that expressive writing works by providing an organizational framework for traumatic memories. Expressive writing pushed people to rearrange their thoughts about their traumatic experiences into more coherent stories. These stories, then, would fit into people's own worldviews. Once this was accomplished, they could "let go" of the trauma, leading to better adjustment.

Josh did an experiment to see if narrative structure was essential to the benefit of expressive writing. Over 100 students were asked to express their deepest thoughts and feelings about the most stressful or traumatic experience of their life, or to engage in emotionally neutral writing. So far, so good, and similar to what many others had done before. The new twist was that one group was asked to write in an explicitly narrative format—they were encouraged to have a clear beginning, middle, and end and to make their writing "story-like." Another group was also asked to express their deepest thoughts and feelings but to do so in a format (essentially a bulleted list, out of temporal order) that deliberately impeded the story-like aspect of a narrative. Both groups produced writing that addressed serious stressful or traumatic topics, and the groups used similar amounts of negative language as assessed by the LIWC. Yet only the group that created a narrative—and told their story—showed any signs of improvement. The fragmented writing group, despite expressing similar amounts of emotion, looked no better than those writing about mundane topics.

Not talking or writing about upsetting experiences, then, can be unhealthy for several reasons. Holding back and not talking about an upsetting experience is bad in and of itself. A deeper problem is that when individuals avoid talking, they fail to translate their thoughts and feelings into language. Without resolving their traumas, they continue to live with them and any negative aftereffects. The health benefits of writing or talking about the traumas, then, are twofold. People reach an understanding of the events and, once this is accomplished, they no longer need to inhibit their talking any further.

Working Memory, Sleep, and Social Connections

We have outlined several components of a general model to explain the effectiveness of written or spoken disclosure. In this chapter so far, most of the processes have been cognitive. That is, they have been describing how emotional disclosure changes the ways we think. Earlier chapters have emphasized other processes that are relevant to the current discussion.

Translating an experience into language, finding meaning in it, and expressing ourselves after actively trying to keep a powerful emotional experience secret are freeing. The overall cognitive changes also result in greater working memory. In other words, once we have put the emotional event into some kind of coherent story that has meaning for us, we no longer need to think about it as much. We are freeing up the mind for other endeavors.

When our mind is no longer working overtime to figure out the complexities of a major upheaval, it can idle in the ways it was designed to do. Instead of sorting through complex emotions and experiences, the traumatized person can now go to sleep more quickly with higher-quality sleep. There should be fewer nightmares, sleeping pills, and bouts of insomnia. Better sleep also facilitates more efficient immune function and cardiovascular activity.

More working memory allows us to pay more attention to the everyday concerns we have always had: What should I fix for dinner? Where did I leave my keys? What is a better way to help my colleagues fix the problem we are all having at work? Why is my good friend so worried about her umbrella? Having sufficient working memory to effectively manage our lives, whether dealing with trivial or more important issues, is at the heart of all of our social relationships.

We are social animals. One of the best predictors of mental and physical health is having a stable and supportive network of friends and family. When we are dealing with major life events, we aren't good and thoughtful friends. Our restricted working memory means we can't listen to others as well. We have more trouble anticipating their problems. Once we have resolved and moved through our own traumas, we can begin connecting with others better.

Putting It All Together: A Disclosure Process Model

Throughout its history, science has struggled with the best way to move forward. In virtually all disciplines, there are the discovery people and the theory people. The discovery people stumble along, find unexpected relationships, and then try to figure out what they mean.

The theory people sit quietly in their offices and try to figure out how the world must work and, once they have a good idea, go out and try to find proof that their ideas are correct. Oftentimes, the discovery and the theory people shake their respective heads at the naiveté of the other group.

In reality, all good scientists have a bit of both discovery and theory inside them.

The original work on emotional disclosure was a pure adventure in discovery. Both authors, however, were generating hypotheses and mini-theories all along to help guide them to the next step. Over the last few decades, the growing number of disclosure researchers have frequently disagreed about why writing works, how powerful the effect really is, and for whom it works best. Through all of this, no single explanation or straightforward theory of disclosure has emerged.

We believe that emotional disclosure and expressive writing very likely work as the result of a cascade of multiple processes that plays out over time. As outlined throughout the book, traumatic experiences immediately disrupt people's daily lives, provoking major emotional upheavals and requiring a rethinking of large parts of their lives. Friendship patterns can quickly alter, and the trauma may strengthen their relationships or undermine them. If people are open and honest with others, they will also begin the process of talking about and working through the trauma.

A more insidious pattern unfolds if people are unable or unwilling to talk openly with others about their emotional upheavals. As we've seen, harboring major secrets tends to isolate the secret keepers, making them less comfortable around their friends from whom they are keeping their secrets. Most problematic, not talking with others means that the people dealing with emotional upheavals are less able to work through their traumas using natural language.

All things being equal, people who have faced major upheavals might benefit more by talking about these issues in detail with persistently supportive friends than by writing. In reality, this often isn't possible. Discussing some emotional upheavals could cause humiliation or might offend or emotionally damage the listeners. It is also quite possible that emotional disclosure could destroy established friendships.

In the weeks or months after a major upheaval, expressive writing can promote healing along several dimensions:

- The mere acknowledgment that the event occurred. Just labeling the actions and emotions starts to produce structure, and creates categories and order that makes sense from the writer's perspective.
- Writing forces additional structure on the experience. A time line is identified and possible causes and effects are explored.
- Multiple perspectives and additional complexities of the experience can be added to the narrative. This can include tying the event to other relevant ones that may have occurred prior, during, or after the experience.
- With continued writing and thinking, perhaps especially so when adopting a self-distanced perspective, a more coherent narrative may emerge—with a clear beginning, middle, and end.
- With repeated telling, the story becomes simpler, more understandable, and more coherent.
- With a more understandable or manageable story, there is less need to continue processing it. Working memory is freed up.
- As people move through the upheaval, they sleep better and have reductions in biological and psychological markers of long-term stress.
- With greater working memory and lower stress levels, people can begin to devote more time to friends and to enjoy higher-quality relationships. Indeed, the boost in social support can help to maintain better health in the future.

Each of the elements that we have outlined has been tested and supported by research. Not all features of this model are part of everyone's story. The components of the disclosure process often work together but can also function independently.

As scientific models go, the disclosure process model is really more of a loose schematic of a series of psychological processes than a tight unitary theory. The components will continue to be tested and debated in the years to come. There are dozens of unanswered questions (and possibly many more). We still don't know what types of writing instructions work best, who is most likely to benefit, which biological processes are most affected by writing, or what the best timing of the writing is.

At this point, many of these unanswered questions can be answered only by the person who tries out expressive writing. In the following chapter, we will point to some of the techniques that have worked in studies. What works in a study may not work for you or your client. You must be your own scientist. If you are interested in expressive writing, experiment on yourself. See what works, drop what doesn't. And come up with some of your own methods that are beneficial for you—some places to start are presented in the next chapter.

CHAPTER 10

Pulling It All Together

RECOMMENDATIONS FOR YOUR USE OF EXPRESSIVE WRITING

The original expressive writing study was based on some hunches. The extent of the original hypothesis was "Hmmm, I wonder if asking people to write about traumas could improve their health." By today's standards, the original experiment had some serious problems, and the size of the benefits was certainly helped along by chance. But it worked. Its effects were etched on the students' faces and, later, what they wrote about being in the study.

Because the first studies worked, researchers and clinicians soon jumped aboard the expressive writing express and started doing similar experiments. It wasn't until at least a decade later that anyone started to seriously question why writing worked or even if the assumptions that we all held were true. In fact, the earlier editions of this book (published in 1990 and 1997) were written just before a new generation of studies was published.

Some of the original assumptions about expressive writing included:

- People had to write about major life traumas
- People had to write about negative experiences that they had kept secret or not divulged in detail to others
- People had to write at least 15 minutes a day for a minimum of three to four times

- Writing probably worked because it stopped people from exerting the effort of active inhibition
- The more that people immersed themselves in their negative feelings, the more likely it was the writing would work
- The writing method was relatively powerful and would work for almost any stress-related mental or physical health problem

These are not outlandish assumptions. Some of them were solidly based on early evidence from the first few studies. But they all appear to be wrong. Although many well-respected clinicians, scientists, and laypeople still hold on to many of them, we are now able to provide a better guide to what works and what doesn't.

This chapter is written for therapists who might want to use expressive writing for their clients, and regular people who might want to use it for themselves. As you read the following pages, you will pick up a recurring theme: Be your own scientist. What works for a group of people in an experiment may or may not work for you. Try different techniques. Keep notes about what makes you feel better or worse. Monitor your behavior while you are experimenting with writing by tracking your sleep, drinking, weight, exercise, and the quality of your relationships and daily mood. Adapt your writing to your context, your needs, and to what works for you.

When Should You Engage in Expressive Writing?

Expressive writing is beneficial in helping to sort out complicated issues. Many of the most complex problems surround powerful emotions related to major life transitions. Almost all of the early writing studies focused on major personal upheavals or traumas. The research evidence now suggests that writing about a wide range of topics can be helpful:

- *Traumatic experiences from the past.* If you find yourself thinking or worrying about an old issue too much, then writing might be beneficial.

- *Current or recent bothersome upheavals.* Writing helps in working through relatively minor problems—a fight with a family member or coworker, failing an exam, anxiety about tackling a new problem, working through a complicated problem at work.

• *Making a life course correction.* Every now and then, it is helpful to stop, stand back, and evaluate how your life is going. Taking a life inventory can help people reevaluate their goals, values, emotions, relationships, and who they are. In the same category would be normal life transitions—either positive or negative. Graduating, falling in love, getting married, and starting a new job are all generally positive experiences but typically require rethinking who we are and where we are going.

• *Stilling the mind.* If you find yourself obsessing about a particular topic or talking about it too much, or if it is impeding your sleep, writing about it can be helpful. As outlined earlier in the book, writing can help people sleep and expand working memory.

When Should You Not Engage in Expressive Writing?

This is a more difficult question to answer because it probably depends on the person and circumstance. The studies that have hinted that expressive writing could be harmful have involved pushing people to engage in emotional processing of events that are overwhelming, are ongoing, or have happened in the previous days or weeks.

This is where you must be your own judge. If, immediately after a terrible experience, you feel you need to write, then write. But if you feel you aren't ready, don't. If you start writing and feel you aren't making progress or you are getting more distressed, stop. Write about less emotional topics. Write about superficial issues. Don't drag yourself through the mud. You are already in the mud.

Other studies have identified some circumstances where writing doesn't seem to help. Note that this is different from those where writing may be harmful or hurtful. For example, in cases of relatively normal (as opposed to traumatic) grief, most studies indicate that writing doesn't help (but also does not hurt) for most people. By the same token, the jury is still out about writing as an aid to caregivers of family members suffering from chronic disease—we simply don't yet know what effect, if any, writing has in this context.

One other situation where writing does not appear to be helpful is when people write about something uncertain that will be happening in the near future. For example, Lillian Nail and her colleagues attempted to use expressive writing for a large group of women who were finishing radiation treatment for breast cancer. Surprisingly, quite a few women who finish medical treatment for breast cancer typically become depressed. This is often attributed to the sudden and dramatic change in the structure and function of their daily routines. Writing in this group had no measurable benefit, perhaps because the women were writing about future outcomes they couldn't know.

Along these lines, Steve Ames at the Mayo Clinic in Orlando, Florida, studied people who were trying to quit smoking. In one study, he had people write before they had actually stopped. In another study, he had them write immediately after stopping. Consistent with Nail's breast cancer study, those writing before stopping had a much vaguer sense of what they would experience once they stopped, and writing was not particularly helpful. When people wrote after they had stopped smoking, the writing intervention was much more successful.

Writing, then, seems to work best when you are trying to come to terms with what has already happened. It appears to be much less effective in preparing you for what might happen in the unknown future.

Is It Necessary to Focus on Traumatic or Negative Experiences?

No. Although writing about emotional upheavals can be helpful, there are many ways to think about them. As described earlier, Laura King and her colleagues found that benefit finding can apparently boost health and mood. Other studies suggest that writing about your most positive experiences in your life can boost health as well.

Even writing about an imaginary trauma can be good for you. One of the most thought-provoking writing experiments of all time was conducted by Melanie Greenberg, Camille Wortman, and Arthur Stone. The researchers found a group of people who had all experienced major upheavals in their lives. About a third of the people were then asked to write about their upheavals in the standard way. Another third wrote about superficial topics. The final third were given the outlines of a personal trauma that they had never experienced. They were then told to *write about this imaginary upheaval as though it had happened to them.*

Think about this for a second. Imagine that you are asked to write a story about learning to drive a car and accidentally running over your pet dog—the dog you have loved more than anything. And your mother has a mild heart attack because of this and continues to blame you for this trauma even though it happened five years ago. Oh, and you don't even drive, have never had a dog, and your mother adores you. We can all imagine writing a powerful essay about the experience as though it happened to us. Most of us have accidentally done something that resulted in great sadness or disappointment. Most of us have deeply hurt a parent.

Writing about an imaginary trauma in a deeply personal way was found to improve people's physical health almost as effectively as writing about their own trauma. This finding should give English teachers and their students some happiness. Writing about emotional topics is more than learning how to put a story together. It is a way for us to learn more about our own emotions, relationships, and thought patterns.

More broadly, the ways we approach a writing topic can have profound effects. Imagine, for example, that you are coping with the divorce of your parents that occurred five years ago. In one scenario, you just write in a way that can help you try to understand the experience; in another you write about the benefits that came from the divorce; in yet another you explore how you could use this experience to become a happier and more successful person in the future. Is it possible that each of these approaches may be helpful?

Deborah Nazarian and Josh did a study to begin to explore just this issue. Interestingly, writing based on each of these approaches proved to be beneficial for participants—but in unexpected ways. These instructions seemed to target multiple processes. Even when asked to focus on one process, instructions often produced changes in *more than one* process. For example, although cognitive-processing instructions directly helped people make sense of the experience, it appears that other instructions (benefit finding, for example) also unintentionally produced greater cognitive processing. Even when we try to focus our writing, there may be some "spillover" effects. Put another way, there may be a common set of responses or processes that are evoked by writing. So, even though we may alter writing instructions to target specific processes we believe are therapeutic, these very

Different Approaches to Expressive Writing

"Standard" expressive writing: Deepest thoughts and feelings about a stressful or traumatic event. Write about the same or different topics over writing sessions.

Cognitive processing: Thoughts and feelings with an attempt to derive more understanding and insight (cognitive processing) regarding a traumatic or stressful event.

Exposure: Deepest thoughts and emotions about the same event across all writing sessions to promote emotional habituation/adaptation.

Benefit finding: Identify an event and then focus on the positive aspects of the experience; this might include a focus on how you have grown or changed as a person due to the event and how you might be better equipped to meet future challenges.

Best possible future self: Think about your life in the future and write about this life as if you have worked hard and succeeded at accomplishing all of your life goals.

specific instructions also elicit a much wider range of responses than those intended to be activated.

How Often, How Long, and How Much Time between Sessions Is Best?

Have you ever wondered why nurses turn very sick patients over every hour or so in the hospital? They do it to prevent bedsores and other complications. But why is it performed once an hour? In the Crimean War, a young nurse, Florence Nightingale, was in charge of a very large group of badly injured soldiers. One night, she was asked to turn each patient over. As it happened, she was the only person on the shift and it took her exactly an hour to turn everyone over before starting over again. Much to the surprise of everyone, her patients did much better than patients under the care of other nurses. Her remarkable and accidental finding changed medical care.

The spread of the expressive writing paradigm was the result of a similar quirk. As noted earlier in the book, the four-day and 15-min-ute-a-day writing method was used in the first experiment and it worked. And the timing was decided by practical rather than any deep theoretical considerations.

Over the last two decades many alternative writing strategies have been tried, and most have worked. Studies have found benefits if people write once, twice, or as many as a dozen times. Writing sessions have ranged from 2 minutes to as long as 30 minutes. The intervals between writing sessions have also fluctuated from 10 minutes to a week or more.

The timing of writing sessions should probably not be random. Writing briefly for as little as two minutes—only once, several times in one day, or on three or four consecutive days—can help people think about, label, and begin to organize their thoughts about topics they may be avoiding. Writing for 10 minutes on three occasions separated by only 10 minutes between sessions can also be beneficial. This intensive writing forces people to process a single experience in great detail.

Although there is relatively little rigorous research on the topic, our intuitive sense is that writing multiple times is better than writing just a single time. Even if the sessions are brief and the space between sessions is as little as two minutes, people report that the between-writing breaks encourage a subtle perspective switch that a single writing session doesn't accomplish.

What Role Does Context or Ritual Play?

Think about the places in modern society where people are most likely to disclose their deepest secrets. Church or other religious institutions, the courtroom, in a therapist's or doctor's office, or around a campfire, on the beach, or even on a late-night drive. All of these are unique settings away from the routines of daily life.

In a clever study by Arden Corter and Keith Petrie, students were asked to write about emotional upheavals in either a stark and brightly lit laboratory room or a more personal, dimly lit and more warmly decorated ("confessional"-style) room. The idea was that the latter, more mysterious, room was more psychologically removed from the students' lives. The more unique and detached setting elicited more emotional and personal stories than the colder laboratory setting.

Is Expressive Writing Effective Only for Certain People?

It's hard to tell. Early research suggested that people more likely to have trouble expressing their emotions were more likely to benefit from writing. Two early studies found that males, people who have trouble labeling their feelings, and people who are hostile or neurotic were particularly responsive to writing. However, these patterns of effects have often not held up or, on occasion, have been found to reverse. At this point, there is no clear picture of which personality dimensions are most likely to respond to expressive writing. In general, then, writing remains effective across a wide range of participant characteristics.

Other projects have attempted to learn whether people from some cultures benefit more from writing than those from other cultures. No clear findings have emerged. Successful writing studies have been reported across multiple countries, languages, and ethnicities. Our belief is that strong emotional and cognitive reactions to important events are likely to be a universal condition, and that people dealing with them can benefit from translating their experiences into narrative language. Such translation may occur through writing, talking with others, prayer, or other narrative and disclosure processes. Having said this, there is reason to suspect that the traditional writing paradigm may be becoming less effective because the idea of writing about stress and worries has become so commonplace—at least in many Western societies. Of course, disclosing emotions has cultural and social meaning; some may see it as okay and acceptable, whereas others do not and see it as inappropriate.

You may be wondering about all the people in these studies who did not get to do the expressive writing. Many studies ask some portion, usually half, of the volunteers to write about emotionally neutral topics to serve as a comparison group to those completing expressive writing. Scientifically, this is an important point as these people are experiencing many of the same things as the expressive writers—they are writing (albeit on different topics), they have to make visits to the research site, are interacting with the researchers, and so forth. Although different studies use different instructions, we have often instructed these volunteers to write about relatively superficial topics such as their activities in the last week, yesterday, and in the upcoming few days. We often label this as a time-management exercise and—thanks to the burgeoning industry that markets time management as a helpful process—our volunteers vigorously engage in these tasks and report them as interesting, valuable, and important. From our perspective, we are happy that such tasks are engaging, but we see no evidence that time management writing improves people's lives.

Putting It into Practice

We want to share with you some of the main points about the writing method that appear to be related to positive health and well-being. Keep in mind that we both approach this largely as researchers and not as therapists, and present general suggestions rather than advice specifically tailored to you. Our recommendations about confronting upsetting events are based on conducting and reading hundreds of research studies, occasional case studies, and the varied experiences that we have had along with a large range of colleagues, students, and collaborators. It is very possible that your writing about your own traumas or upsetting feelings may not be immediately helpful. If this happens, you should be your own researcher. Experiment with different topics and approaches. Something may work for you in resolving your own conflicts that may not work for anyone else. With these caveats in mind, here are some general guidelines to use, followed by some questions frequently asked about the writing method. You may have already started to explore writing with some of the exercises in earlier chapters; if so, some of this will be familiar, but we will present additional details.

GETTING READY TO WRITE

Find a time and place where you won't be disturbed. Ideally, pick a time at the end of your workday or in the evening when you know things will be calm and quiet. Promise yourself that you will write for a minimum of 15 minutes a day for at least three or four consecutive days, or a fixed day and time for several weeks (for example, every Thursday evening for this month). Once you begin writing, write continuously. Don't worry about spelling or grammar. If you run out of things to write about, just repeat what you have already written. You can write longhand or you can type on a computer. If you are unable to write, you can also talk into a tape recorder. You can write about the same thing on all days of writing or you can write about something different each day. It is entirely up to you.

Detailed Expressive Writing Instructions

Over the next four days, I want you to write about your deepest emotions and thoughts about the most upsetting experience in your life. Really let go and explore your feelings and thoughts about it. In your writing, you might tie this experience to your childhood, your relationship with your parents, people you have loved or love now, or even your career. How is this experience related to who you would like to become, who you have been in the past, or who you are now?

Many people have not had a single traumatic experience, but all of us have had major conflicts or stressors in our lives, and you can write about them as well. You can write about the same issue every day or a series of different issues. Whatever you choose to write about, however, it is critical that you really let go and explore your very deepest emotions and thoughts.

Warning: Many people report that after writing, they sometimes feel somewhat sad or depressed. As with seeing a sad movie, this typically goes away in a couple of hours. If you find that you are getting extremely upset about a writing topic, simply stop writing or change topics.

WHAT SHOULD YOUR WRITING TOPIC BE?

It is not necessary to write about the most traumatic experience of your life. It may be more useful to focus on those issues that you are currently living with. You can also write about topics from the distant past that you are still living with. If you find yourself thinking or dreaming about an event or experience too much of the time, writing about it can help to resolve it in your mind. By the same token, if there has been something that you would like to tell others but you can't for fear of embarrassment or punishment, it may be helpful to express it on paper.

Whatever your topic, it is critical to explore both the objective experience (i.e., what happened) and your feelings about it. Really let go and write about your very deepest emotions. *What* do you feel about it and *why* do you feel that way? How does it influence your life? Your relationships? Your goals and dreams?

WHEN AND WHERE SHOULD YOU WRITE?

Write whenever you want or whenever you feel you need to. The evidence suggests that writing about significant experiences does not need to be done that frequently. Although many people write every day in diaries, most of the entries do not grapple with fundamental psychological issues. Also be attentive to *too* much writing. Don't use writing as a substitute for action or as some other type of avoidance strategy. Moderation in all things includes putting your thoughts and feelings onto paper.

Where you write depends on your circumstances. Some studies suggest that a more unusual or unique setting may be better. Most important is to try to find a room where you will not be interrupted or bothered by unwanted sounds, sights, or smells.

WHAT SHOULD YOU DO WITH WHAT YOU HAVE WRITTEN?

Anonymity is important in our experiments, and we generally advocate it for your own writing as well. In many cases, it is wise to plan to keep what you have written to yourself—this will help you be completely honest with yourself in your writing. You might even destroy it when you're finished (although many people find this hard to do). Planning to show your writing to someone can change your mind-set while writing. For example, if you would secretly like your lover to read your deepest thoughts and feelings, you will orient your writing to your lover rather than to yourself. From a health perspective, you will be better off making yourself the audience. In that way, you won't have to rationalize or justify yourself in writing to suit the perspective of another person. Some people keep their samples and edit them over time, gradually changing their writing from day to day. Others simply keep them and return to reread them over and over again to see how they have changed over time.

WHAT IF YOU HATE TO WRITE—IS THERE A SUBSTITUTE?

A number of studies have compared writing with all kinds of other disclosure modalities—most commonly talking (e.g., into a recording device). Most studies find that, as long as the broad approach is otherwise similar, different modalities are largely comparable in effectiveness. Our bias is that longhand writing makes a bit more sense, since you need only paper and pen and a quiet spot to disclose feelings. Writing also slows you down a bit, helping you tackle one aspect at a time of what are often complicated and emotionally challenging experiences. Talking also requires a recorder and somewhere to talk aloud where you won't be heard (or have to worry about being heard). With that said, find the approach that you are most comfortable with and that you will be able to fully commit to.

Whether writing or talking is a more comfortable medium for you, remember that letting go and disclosing intimate parts of yourself and your experiences may take some practice. If you have never written or talked about your thoughts and feelings, you may find doing so particularly awkward at first. If so, just relax and practice. Write or talk continuously for a set amount of time, typically at least 15 to 20 minutes. No one is evaluating you.

WHAT CAN YOU EXPECT TO FEEL DURING AND AFTER WRITING?

You may feel sad or a little depressed immediately after writing. These negative feelings usually dissipate within an hour or so. In rare cases, they may last for a day or two. The overwhelming majority of our volunteers, however, report feelings of relief, happiness, and contentment soon after the writing studies are concluded.

CODA

Disclosing your deepest thoughts and feelings through writing or talking is not a panacea, not a magical cure-all that will make all your troubles and aches go away. If you are deeply struggling to deal with trauma or with an illness, writing should not be used as a substitute or replacement for other psychological or medical treatment. Rather, writing serves you best as a form of ongoing preventive maintenance. If you are coping with death, divorce, trauma, or other tragedy, you will very likely not feel instantly better after writing. You should, however, have a better understanding of your feelings and emotions as well as the objective situation that you are in. In other words, writing should give you a little distance and, hopefully, enhanced perspective on your life. Over time, that may very well help you feel better.

Notes

Chapter 1

PAGE 8: Psychological and social influences on health and well-being:
There are many fields that study mind–body relationships, or the influence
of thoughts, feelings, and behaviors on health—including health psychology (which primarily focuses on intrapsychic processes, such as thoughts
and emotions) and behavioral medicine (a bit more focused on behavioral
influences on health). There are many superb books that provide a nice
introduction to these issues—one of our favorites is Shelley Taylor's *Health
Psychology*. Another is Robert Sapolsky's *Why Zebras Don't Get Ulcers*.

Chapter 2

PAGE 17: The original expressive writing study: The experiment (Pennebaker & Beall, 1986) was actually more complex than portrayed in the
text. There were three experimental conditions and a control group. The
condition of most relevance is described in the text. The other two conditions were having people write about their emotions but include no facts
about the trauma and having people write just about the facts but not
their emotions. Neither of these latter conditions produced any benefit to
the student writers. Overall, there were only 46 students in the experiment. Looking back today and knowing how modest the expressive writing results generally are, it was dumb luck that the study came out as
beautifully as it did.

Chapter 3

PAGE 27: Talking about a trauma is a natural human response: When it comes to disclosing strong emotional experiences, people have different natural tendencies. Some are clearly more willing—and even strongly desire—to disclose. In contrast, others are more likely to keep things to themselves, and will naturally desire to disclose—or actually disclose— less frequently.

PAGE 34: Physiological activation: The idea of different autonomic patterns being linked to different psychological states has a long history in the field of psychophysiology. Three pioneers in this world have been John Lacey, Paul Obrist, and Don Fowles. The distinction between the cardiovascular (e.g., heart rate and blood pressure) and electrodermal systems (e.g., skin conductance) was first suggested by Fowles in 1982. More recent work on heart rate variability (HRV) points to its link to emotional expression and expressive writing.

PAGE 38: The powerful effects of emotional processing: Daniel Goleman's (1995) book *Emotional Intelligence* paints a thoughtful portrait of emotion processing in psychotherapy.

PAGE 39: New research on how our brains process and shape social interactions: Matthew Lieberman, a professor at the University of California, Los Angeles, has presented an excellent exploration of new research in social neuroscience in his 2014 book *Social: Why Our Brains Are Wired to Connect*.

Chapter 4

PAGE 55: Extending these findings: Another study by Walker and colleagues in 1999 sought to examine the feasibility of using emotional expression to help cancer patients improve psychosocial health outcomes. Although their findings did not show significant improvements in psychosocial health outcomes, some of the main themes that arose from the written work show that these women were having similar issues surrounding communication, the possibility of recurrence, and their own health behaviors, findings that could aid medical professionals in future research.

PAGE 57: Other effects of expressive writing on patients: In addition, the broader effect of expressive writing on physical outcomes has been demonstrated by faster wound healing in healthy older adults (Koschwanez et al., 2013) and healthy male volunteers (Weinman, Ebrecht, Scott, Walburn, & Dyson, 2008) and fewer complications and lower diastolic blood pressure after myocardial infarction (Willmott, Harris, Gellaitry, Cooper, & Horne, 2011).

PAGE 58: The effects of writing on related domains: The effects of expressive writing on mental health outcomes have been mixed, but promising in some areas. As we saw from Josh's early meta-analysis of expressive writing, early work showed positive effects on symptoms of depression, anxiety, and academic performance. Later related work has replicated and extended academically relevant findings in student groups, showing that expressive writing results in greater working memory capacity (Klein & Boals, 2001b; Yogo & Fujihara, 2008), greater improvements in grade-point average (Lumley & Provenzano, 2003), and higher graduate entrance exam scores (Frattaroli, Thomas, & Lyubomirsky, 2011).

PAGE 60: Writing may help reduce mental distress: Some evidence for the benefit of expressive writing on depression and general distress has also been shown. For example, among university students, expressive writing led to fewer depressive symptoms six months after writing (Gortner, Rude, & Pennebaker, 2006). Expressive writing also has been shown to protect students against upsetting intrusive or unwanted thoughts about stressful experiences (Lepore, 1997) and from rumination about such experiences (Sloan, Marx, Epstein, & Dobbs, 2008).

PAGE 60: The emerging field of exploring writing to help manage PTSD: In one small study, 22 participants with PTSD were instructed to write about the most stressful aspects of their illness. Expressive writing resulted in less severity and avoidance of symptoms (Bernard, Jackson, & Jones, 2006). Other small studies have been inconclusive as to the benefits of writing, particularly when used in conjunction with other forms of disclosure (e.g., both writing and talking with others about trauma).

PAGE 64: Expressive writing may be clinically useful, efficient, and cost-effective: Interest in expressive writing has persisted since the mid-1980s, in part due to its potential clinical utility. The intervention itself is brief, low cost, and easily administered when compared to other approaches. As such, expressive writing has been seen as a potentially useful adjunct to traditional psychotherapy methods. For example, Mosher and colleagues (2012) showed that cancer patients who engaged in expressive writing (vs. control writing) were more likely to access mental health services; thus, expressive writing may help patients identify areas of need or otherwise prepare them to seek beneficial resources. Graf, Guadiano, and Geller (2008) also demonstrated that using expressive writing exercises as homework between psychotherapy sessions (vs. control writing homework) led to greater progress in therapy and larger reductions in symptoms of depression and anxiety. Similar benefits were observed among psychotherapy clients whose partners had engaged in extramarital affairs (Gordon, Baucom, & Snyder, 2007).

Cummings and colleagues (2014) also describe and illustrate several advantages of expressive writing as part of clinical intervention. Initially, this type of writing can be used for self-monitoring and increasing awareness of personal experiences, which can lead into its use for promoting exposure and cognitive processing. As therapy progresses, expressive writing can aid in tracking symptom changes and improving the therapeutic alliance. As Cummings and others have noted, however, incorporating expressive writing into psychotherapy should be carefully considered. As this type of writing tends to increase immediate distress (Smyth, 1998), therapists should prepare clients for this experience and discuss tools for managing such distress. The optimal number or length of sessions may differ between clients, and some clients may benefit from receiving feedback whereas others may wish to keep their written narratives private (opting to summarize them during therapy sessions). Clients who encounter barriers to handwriting narratives (such as physical disability or literacy issues) also could type or speak into an audio recorder. The flexibility in session parameters, including the specific instructions used, allows clinicians to adapt expressive writing to particular client needs.

Additional issues regarding when and how best to use expressive writing are explored in Chapter 10.

PAGE 64: Expressive writing in the context of stigma: There has also been interest in the use of expressive writing with members of stigmatized or marginalized groups (e.g., ethnic minority, LGBT [lesbian, gay, bisexual, and transgender], and those diagnosed with certain illnesses), as members of these groups often inhibit or avoid disclosure about their group status. Thus, expressive writing may be particularly useful for identifying and managing thoughts and feelings related to status that they feel unwilling or unable to discuss freely with others. Expressive writing about the stress related to the experience of gay male college students led to more openness about sexual orientation three months later (Pachankis & Goldfried, 2010). Similarly, expressive writing has produced other psychological benefits among HIV-positive adults high in "cognitive adaptability" (Wagner, Hilker, Hepworth, & Wallston, 2010) and gay women who were less open (versus more) about their sexuality prior to writing (Lewis et al., 2005).

PAGE 64: Writing and health behaviors: Although there is great inconsistency in relating expressive writing to health behaviors, much of that work is based on secondary assessments of health behaviors (such as diet, smoking, exercise) included in other studies. Another line of work has used expressive writing as an adjunct to other methods but has directly targeted substance use outcomes. A study on young adult smokers found that expressive writing, in addition to a brief cessation session, resulted in higher abstinence rates from smoking for a longer period of time than just the cessation session group (Ames et al., 2007). Ames and colleagues have published the first investigation on the efficacy and feasibility of an intervention using expressive writing for smoking cessation. Using a brief intervention and adjunct expressive writing task, they found little difference between the group that had only the brief cessation training compared to the group that had expressive writing and cessation training. This could be due to a few factors, such as the high percentage of participants who were already abstaining from tobacco at baseline, length of treatment, and the possibility of participants not truly self-reflecting in their writing.

PAGE 64: Improvements in health and well-being through our care-seeking behavior: Another domain of interest has been the effect of expressive writing on health care utilization. As with the effects on students' utilization of campus health care services described earlier, later tests of expressive writing showed fewer infirmary visits among prison inmates (Richards, Beall, Seagal, & Pennebaker, 2000) and fewer medical visits by patients with prostate cancer (Rosenberg et al., 2002), breast cancer (Stanton et al., 2002), or fibromyalgia (Gillis, Lumley, Mosley-Williams, Leisen, & Roehrs, 2006) following expressive writing.

Researchers also examined utilization among groups selected for psychological distress, who may be more likely to access medical or mental health care than the general population. Findings in this area are mixed: Expressive writing led to decreased utilization in students affected by close others committing suicide (Kovac & Range, 2000) or a history of trauma (Deters & Range, 2003). Yet among bereaved individuals, there was either no effect (Range, Kovac, & Marion, 2000) or an increase in utilization after expressive writing (Stroebe, Stroebe, Schut, Zech, & van den Bout, 2002). Undergraduates who reported many physical symptoms also showed greater utilization after expressive writing (Lumley, Leegstra, Provenzano, & Warren, 1999).

A meta-analysis of the effects of expressive writing on health care utilization (Harris, 2006) showed that, overall, there were significant (but small) reductions in utilization among healthy and medical samples. In psychiatric samples, utilization did not differ between expressive writing and control writing groups. Importantly, Harris (2006) notes that the meaning of differences or change in health care utilization requires examination on a case-by-case basis. For example, a reduction for those "overutilizing" services might be positive, whereas an increase for some avoiding health care systems would be beneficial. As such, it is not readily known whether decreased utilization is a desirable outcome for each person. The benefit of expressive writing for health care utilization is thus context and person specific.

Finally, to present another approach, another study attempted to train physicians to elicit disclosure from patients. Patients who were frequent visitors of general medical practice due to somatic symptoms were visited by trained "disclosure doctors" with whom they discussed emotionally significant experiences. The disclosure intervention was not effective— there were no differences between the treatment group and the group that received standard care (Schilte et al., 2001). It is not clear if this is due to the interpersonal nature of the disclosure, something about the patients selected, the choice of physicians to disclose to (who may, for instance, have "reverted" to medical care advice), or other factors.

Chapter 5

PAGE 66: Notes and learning: Interestingly, students who take "summarized" notes versus verbatim notes comprehend material better. It appears that summarized note taking fosters the process of transforming the information into something meaningful and integrating new information with previously known information (Hagen, Braasch, & Braten, 2014).

PAGE 75: Advent of the computer and Internet: In today's technology-driven world, the Internet has proven a potentially useful tool for people to disclose their thoughts and emotions. Twitter, Instagram, Facebook, and other social networking sites provide tremendous opportunities for written (and other) disclosure. As Internet access has become more and more prevalent, there have been efforts to examine disclosure interventions delivered in an online format (particularly as a way to reach individuals unwilling or unable to seek interpersonal therapy). One of the first studies of this type was conducted in 2003 by Alfred Lange and his colleagues in Amsterdam, the Netherlands. In an online written disclosure therapy study for traumatized individuals, symptoms of PTSD (intrusions, avoidance, and general psychopathology) improved significantly compared following online disclosure (Lange et al., 2003).

The Internet as a mode to explore writing interventions offers privacy and is less expensive than traditional face-to-face studies. For instance, Bond and Pennebaker (2012) conducted an online writing intervention to determine whether directed feedback would change the way people used personal pronouns and improve mood. A more recent study by Hannah Stockton and her colleagues (2014) examined the effects of Internet-based ("online") intervention designed to facilitate disclosure about traumatic experiences on posttraumatic growth. Those assigned to disclose, relative to those in an emotionally neutral comparison condition, showed enhanced posttraumatic growth over two months. These researchers also looked at the language used in the essays typed online—the more frequent use of words related to insight and understanding (presumably related to making sense of things, or meaning making) was associated with an increase in posttraumatic growth. A plethora of other electronic interventions (Baikie, Geerligs, & Wilhelm, 2012; Halpert, Rybin, & Doros, 2010; Hirai, Skidmore, Clum, & Dolma, 2012) show how such changes (and many more not delineated here) may be altering the nature and meaning of expressive writing. This is clearly an area that will require much more study and examination.

Chapter 6

PAGE 83: What is rumination: Rumination is typically defined as a style of repetitive cognitions (thoughts) that focus the depressed individual's attention on his or her symptoms, the potential causes and consequences of those symptoms, but in nonproductive ways. Individuals who suppress thoughts appear somewhat more likely to be ruminators. Both require cognitive effort and may represent incomplete cognitive processing or disrupted/ineffective efforts to "make sense" of experiences. As more effort is used to suppress thoughts, the thoughts become more and more accessible. Rumination can also predict depressive episodes in some individuals, and formerly depressed individuals display high rates of rumination and thought suppression.

PAGE 84: Ironic process theory: Wegner's ironic process theory says that "intentional operating processes" of thought suppression are effortful; in other words, intentionally trying to suppress thoughts is difficult. Many people, for example, will try to suppress a thought by distracting themselves by focusing on some object in immediate sight. Such strategies, however, do not typically work—the target distractor object tends to not hold our attention long, and our minds tend to return to the original (suppressed) thought relatively quickly. Ultimately then, these distractions may remind the individual of the suppressed thought. Wegner also proposes that an "ironic monitoring process" operating in the background of our consciousness allows us to unconsciously monitor for unwanted thoughts and simply alerts the intentional operating process when the unwanted thought occurs that a distraction is needed (Wenzlaff & Wegner, 2000).

PAGE 84: Accepting the unacceptable: The interested reader is again encouraged to look at Brené Brown's work. Several of her books (e.g., *The Gifts of Imperfection*; *Daring Greatly*) extend this concept and apply it to everyday living. She suggests that letting go of who you *think* you ought to be will help you understand, accept, and embrace who you actually are. In doing this, she believes, you can live a life with more joy, compassion, and gratitude.

PAGE 85: Thought cycles that people coping with PTSD struggle with: There are some risk factors for the development of posttraumatic symptoms or even PTSD following exposure to traumatic events or experiences. Individuals who are highly reactive to novel stimuli, highly anxious, avoidant, and self-blaming, or high in hypnotic ability, may be particularly susceptible to traumatic experiences. Similarly, the more extreme the trauma and the longer the time over which it lasts, the higher the incidence of PTSD (e.g., Breslau, Chilcoat, Kessler, & Davis, 1999). It is also generally agreed that people most prone to PTSD have had a history of depression, trauma, and other PTSD episodes in the past even prior to their most recent traumatic experience (Cabrera, Hoge, Bliese, Castro, & Messer, 2007).

PAGE 90: The benefits of mindfulness: There are now hundreds of books and articles on topics related to mindfulness, some that examine the systematic practices of mindfulness and meditation, others that apply the general ideas and concepts to specific tasks (work, relationships, etc.) or daily life. Does mindfulness work? Accumulating evidence suggests that, at least among those who diligently practice the techniques and successfully integrate them into daily life, mindfulness and meditative practices can have potent health and well-being benefits. Much of the clinical application and research, as noted in the main text, emerged from the early work of Kabat-Zinn and has used variations of mindfulness-based stress reduction; he wrote an excellent summary of the current state and future possibilities of mindfulness-based interventions that is an excellent orientation to the broader evidence (Kabat-Zinn, 2003). A review and meta-analysis of studies that have used mindfulness-based stress reduction on healthy people showed that it was able to aid in multiple health outcomes, including reducing ruminative thoughts and anxiety levels, increasing empathy, and increasing self-compassion (Chiesa & Serretti, 2009). Finally, an intriguing study by Moore and colleagues examined whether disclosure could improve mindfulness, mental health, and experiential avoidance. Narrative disclosure did not itself improve outcomes, but those individuals who showed enhanced mindfulness also showed improved mental health (Moore, Brody, & Dierberger, 2009).

PAGE 93: Disclosure and sleep: There is growing evidence that expressive writing can help with a broad array of sleep-related processes, even when the writing is not specifically targeted at sleep. For instance, a study conducted by Danielle Arigo and Josh found that an expressive writing intervention for college women—even though it was largely focused on helping the young women with body image dissatisfaction—led to improved sleep (Arigo & Smyth, 2012). Another study used expressive writing to help cancer patients diagnosed with renal cell carcinoma. Separate from outcomes related to adjustment to the cancer, the patients reported less sleep disturbance after writing when compared to a group of patients who did not write (de Moor et al., 2002). These kinds of findings continue to accrue—expressive writing has further been related to shorter sleep onset latency (i.e., how long it takes to fall asleep once going to bed), less arousal prior to trying to sleep, and reduced symptoms of insomnia (Gortner et al., 2006; Harvey & Farrell, 2003; Mooney, Espie, & Broomfield, 2009).

Chapter 7

PAGE 99: Understanding loss and bereavement: A prominent researcher in this area, George Bonanno, has extensively studied this issue—one line of work examines responses to bereavement (typically the death of a spouse). Bonanno suggests that the ways people grieve are highly dependent on the ways they view their loss as it relates to other issues in their lives. He has identified at least five different grief trajectories: common grief, chronic grief, chronic depression, depression followed by improvement, and resilience. People with chronic grief typically felt that their loss caused a major upheaval in all parts of their lives. Those with chronic depression viewed the death of their spouse as simply exacerbating their depressed state. Those who appeared resilient and those who were only temporarily depressed both appeared to be healthy and not to be struggling or denying/avoiding the loss.

PAGE 103: What *does* work after a traumatic experience?: The short answer is that we still don't really know. One interesting line of work suggests that, at least in some cases, approaches that focus on building and enhancing a narrative surrounding the trauma may be particularly useful. For instance, in a study of children following disaster, a trauma narrative approach was slightly better than a coping training (Salloum & Overstreet, 2012).

PAGE 104: Bereavement and subsequent health: Bereaved individuals are at risk for early mortality, physical health symptoms (headaches, indigestion), higher medication use, and higher rates of disability. Acute suffering is common; however, for some these symptoms can become clinically relevant (i.e., develop into clinical depression, PTSD, etc.; Stroebe, Schut, & Stroebe, 2007). Research suggests that although thinking about the loss may often be a necessary process to resolve the stress associated with loss, ongoing negative psychological intrusions are harmful. Thus, intervening in the process of cognitive processing may help to prevent the development of chronic or clinical distress (Lepore & Greenberg, 2002).

PAGE 105: Expressive writing for traumatized children and adolescents: In a provocative study of Afghani children and adolescents bereaved after disaster, Kalantari, Yule, Dyregrov, Neshatdoost, & Ahmadi (2012) found that a variant of expressive writing—"Writing for Recovery"—was found to be an effective group intervention.

PAGE 106: Other issues involving couples or dyads: Expressing emotion, including through writing, about relationship distress and trauma may help couples "create a shared cognitive schema essential to intimacy and trust." Extramarital affairs, for example, may cause one partner's view of the world to shift (e.g., that they no longer have a trustworthy partner who values them), causing depression, distress, and shame. The expressive writing paradigm has been applied to couple therapy for dealing with affairs in the form of letter writing. It may help couples build a new base and create new expectations/assumptions about their relationship, promoting more positive interactions and less distress, depression, and anger (Snyder, Gordon, & Baucom, 2004).

PAGE 106: Understanding and moving beyond grief: There are a number of good books on this topic. If you are interested in more detail, we suggest Parkes, C. M. (2008). *Love and Loss: The Roots of Grief and Its Complications*. London & New York: Routledge.

Chapter 8

PAGE 116: Secrets, sharing, and friendship: This viewpoint asserts that the process of disclosure involves (1) a decision to disclose in an attempt to reach a desired goal (e.g., enhanced relationship intimacy), (2) the actual communication between disclosure and confidant, (3) processes that elicit relationship changes (changes in social support, inhibition, and social information), and (4) feedback loops (a disclosure event will impact subsequent events by increasing or decreasing the capacity and willingness of the discloser to disclose). Also, as noted, disclosure events are a component of "stigma management"—that is, by participating in one disclosure event, individuals can "test the water" and determine reactions/cope with consequences. The outcome of these probes will determine whether future disclosure events occur.

PAGE 121: Extramarital affairs: The discovery of an extramarital affair often has devastating effects on a marriage. Gordon and colleagues explored the use of an integrative treatment, including a letter-writing-based emotional disclosure component, to enhance the chance of positive recovery for couples going through an affair issue. Couples reported less marital distress and greater forgiveness for the offense at the end of treatment compared to when they began.

PAGE 123: Friends and secrets: Jamie found when examining data from a large sample of corporate employees, that people with large social support networks who kept a big secret about a major trauma had more health problems than people who had small social support networks. Presumably, holding back a big secret is far more work for people with lots of friends.

PAGE 129: Stress and infectious disease: As an interesting aside, research psychologist Sheldon Cohen and his colleagues at Carnegie Mellon University have convincingly demonstrated through a series of elegant studies that this supposition is quite true—psychological stress can meaningfully increase the likelihood of becoming ill, and the severity of illness, after exposure to the common cold virus.

Chapter 9

PAGE 138: Trying to make sense of trauma: A fascinating paper by Alison Holman and colleagues on a broad array of trauma survivors (adult victims of childhood incest, Vietnam War veterans, and residents of two southern California communities devastated by fire) shows that a past temporal orientation—focusing attention on prior life trauma—was associated with increased levels of psychological distress many years after the trauma had passed. Importantly, the negative effect of past temporal orientation was present even when accounting for other factors known to impact persistent distress, including self-reported rumination. This finding suggests that a general tendency to focus on the past can be harmful above and beyond ruminating about specific (negative) events, perhaps by impeding one's capacity to make sense of the experience and move forward.

PAGE 142: Do we need to process and understand all trauma?: It is also the case that in some circumstances such processing may not be necessary and many people don't spend time "figuring out" the trauma and nonetheless cope quite well.

PAGE 148: Other mediums of expression: Over the years, both Jamie and Josh have brought people into the lab and hooked them up to physiological monitors (e.g., to measure heart rate, blood pressure, and skin conductance). Sometimes they are asked to sing. Sometimes to draw, or even dance. Generally, the more comfortable people are with the medium, the more they tend to relax (as measured by the biological data) when expressing themselves through singing or drawing. But people are typically quite willing to express themselves regardless of the medium.

PAGE 148: Reading literature and health: There is also some fascinating evidence that people who read classic literature become healthier and more socially skilled (Kidd & Castano, 2013); see also a nice story on this topic at *http://well.blogs.nytimes.com/2013/10/03/i-know-how-youre-feeling-i-read-chekhov.*

PAGE 149: More on dance and movement therapy: The project conducted by Anne Krantz is consistent with recent findings indicating that dance or movement therapies can improve breast cancer patients' quality of life, relieve depression and psychological distress, and improve balance and coordination in Parkinson's disease and heart failure patients. In fact, dance therapy has also been shown to reduce pain and symptoms among people with advanced cancer. (See also Selman, Williams, & Simms, 2012.)

PAGE 156: The components of the disclosure process: As should be clear from the text so far, there is evidence consistent with many different explanations for how or why disclosure is helpful. The exact nature of how disclosure "works" is explained differently from therapist to therapist or researcher to researcher. Many theories posit that disclosure, whether through verbal communication or writing, is beneficial because of the cognitive processing that it facilitates. For example, the exposure theory of experimental disclosure suggests that experimental disclosure is similar to exposure therapy, used most commonly to treat phobias and PTSD. The idea is that, in time, disclosure leads to a reduction in negative thoughts and feelings associated with the event in question. A different theory, the social cognitive processing theory advanced by Stephen Lepore (2001) and others, states that individuals must cognitively process their emotions and thoughts *with others* in order to adjust to stressful events or traumatic experiences. That is, others can help us better understand, interpret, and cope with traumatic experiences and the feelings and thoughts we have about those experiences (although sometimes disclosing to others can cause more harm than good). The social integration model says disclosure may change how people interact with friends and family, which could influence health. Several studies have found that those who participated in an experimental disclosure exercise were more likely to discuss with others the traumatic experience from their past, and were more likely to report receiving social support than were people who did not disclose.

Bibliography

Altman, I., & Taylor, D. A. (1973). *Social Penetration: The Development of Interpersonal Relationships*. New York: Holt.

Ames, S. C., Patten, C. A., Offord, K. P., Pennebaker, J. W., Croghan, I. T., Tri, D. M., et al. (2005). Expressive writing intervention for young adult cigarette smokers. *Journal of Clinical Psychology, 61*(12), 1555–1570.

Ames, S. C., Patten, C. A., Werch, C. E., Schroeder, D. R., Stevens, S. R., Fredrickson, P. A., et al. (2007). Expressive writing as a smoking cessation treatment adjunct for young adult smokers. *Nicotine and Tobacco Research, 9*(2), 185–194.

Archer, S., Buxton, S., & Sheffield, D. (2014). The effect of creative psychological interventions on psychological outcomes for adult cancer patients: A systematic review of randomised controlled trials. *Psycho-Oncology, 24*(1), 1–10.

Arden-Close, E., Gidron, Y., Bayne, L., & Moss-Morris, R. (2013). Written emotional disclosure for women with ovarian cancer and their partners: Randomized controlled trial. *Psycho-Oncology, 22*(10), 2262–2269.

Arigo, D., & Smyth, J. M. (2012). The benefits of expressive writing on sleep difficulty and appearance concerns for college women. *Psychology and Health, 27*(2), 210–226.

Baikie, K. A., Geerligs, L., & Wilhelm, K. (2012). Expressive writing and positive writing for participants with mood disorders: An online randomized controlled trial. *Journal of Affective Disorders, 136*(3), 310–319.

Baikie, K. A., & Wilhelm, K. (2005). Emotional and physical benefits of expressive writing. *Advances in Psychiatric Treatment, 11*(5), 338–346.

Bangert-Drowns, R. L., Hurley, M. M., & Wilkinson, B. (2004). The effects of school-based writing-to-learn interventions on academic achievement: A meta-analysis. *Review of Educational, 74*(1), 29–58.

Barak, A., Hen, L., Boniel-Nissim, M., & Shapira, N. (2008). A comprehensive review and a meta-analysis of the effectiveness of Internet-based psychotherapeutic interventions. *Journal of Technology in Human Services, 26*(2/4), 109–160.

Barclay, L. J., & Skarlicki, D. P. (2009). Healing the wounds of organizational injustice: Examining the benefits of expressive writing. *Journal of Applied Psychology, 94*(2), 511.

Belanoff, P., Elbow, P., & Fontaine, S. I. (Eds.). (1991). *Nothing Begins with N: New Investigations of Freewriting.* Carbondale: Southern Illinois Press.

Bernard, M., Jackson, C., & Jones, C. (2006). Written emotional disclosure following first episode psychosis: Effects on symptoms of PTSD. *British Journal of Clinical Psychology, 45*, 403–415.

Bonanno, G. A. (2005). Resilience in the face of potential trauma. *Current Directions in Psychological Science, 14*(3), 135–138.

Bonnano, G. A., & Mancini, A. D. (2008). The human capacity to thrive in the face of potential trauma. *Pediatrics, 121*(2), 369–375.

Bonanno, G. A., Westphal, M., & Mancini, A. D. (2011). Resilience to loss and potential trauma. *Annual Review of Clinical Psychology, 7*, 511–535.

Bonanno, G. A., Wortman, C. B., Lehman, D. R., Tweed, R. G., Haring, M., Sonnega, J., et al. (2002). Resilience to loss and chronic grief: A prospective study from preloss to 18-months postloss. *Journal of Personality and Social Psychology, 83*(5), 1150.

Bonanno, G. A., Wortman, C. B., & Nesse, R. M. (2004). Prospective patterns of resilience and maladjustment during widowhood. *Psychology and Aging, 19*(2), 260.

Bond, M., & Pennebaker, J. W. (2012). Automated computer-based feedback in expressive writing. *Computers in Human Behavior, 28*(3), 1014–1018.

Boniel-Nissim, M., & Barak, A. (2012). The Internet to the aid of lonely adolescents: The therapeutic value of blog writing. *Mifgash Le'Avoda Socialit Chinuchit, 34*, 9–30.

Bowlby, J. (1958). The nature of the child's tie to his mother. *International Journal of Psycho-Analysis, 39*(5), 350–373.

Breslau, N., Chilcoat, H. D., Kessler, R. C., & Davis, G. C. (1999). Previous exposure to trauma and PTSD effects of subsequent trauma: Results from the Detroit area survey of trauma. *American Journal of Psychiatry, 156*, 902–907.

Breuer, J., & Freud, S. (1895/1966). *Studies in Hysteria.* New York: Avon Press.

Broderick, J. E., Junghaenel, D. U., & Schwartz, J. E. (2005). Written emotional expression produces health benefits in fibromyalgia patients. *Psychosomatic Medicine, 67*(2), 326–334.

Broderick, J. E., Stone, A. A., Smyth, J. M., & Kaell, A. T. (2004). The feasibility and effectiveness of an expressive writing intervention for rheumatoid arthritis via home-based videotaped instruction. *Annals of Behavioral Medicine, 27*(1), 50–59.

Brown, B. (2010). *The Gifts of Imperfection: Let Go of Who You Think You Are Supposed to Be and Embrace Who You Are.* Center City, MN: Hazelden.

Brown, B. (2012). *Daring Greatly: How the Courage to Be Vulnerable Transforms the Way We Live, Love, Parent, and Lead.* New York: Avery.

Cabrera, O. A., Hoge, C. W., Bliese, P. D., Castro, C. A., & Messer, S. C. (2007). Childhood adversity and combat as predictors of depression and posttraumatic stress in deployed troops. *American Journal of Preventative Medicine, 33,* 77–82.

Cameron, L. D., & Nicholls, G. (1998). Expression of stressful experiences through writing: Effects of a self-regulation manipulation for pessimists and optimists. *Health Psychology, 17*(1), 84.

Carmack, C. L., Basen-Engquist, K., Yuan, Y., Greisinger, A., Rodriguez-Bigas, M., Wolff, R. A., et al. (2011). Feasibility of an expressive disclosure group intervention for post-treatment colorectal cancer patients. *Cancer, 117,* 4993–5002.

Chaudoir, S. R., & Fisher, J. D. (2010). The disclosure process model: Understanding disclosure decision making and postdisclosure outcomes among people living with a concealable stigmatized identity. *Psychological Bulletin, 136*(2), 236–256.

Chiesa, A., & Serretti, A. (2009). Mindfulness-based stress reduction for stress management in healthy people: A review and meta-analysis. *Journal of Alternative and Complementary Medicine, 15*(5), 593–600.

Chung, C. K., & Pennebaker, J. W. (2008). Variations in spacing of expressive writing sessions. *British Journal of Health Psychology, 13,* 15–21.

Cobb, S. (1976). Social support as a moderator of life stress. *Psychosomatic Medicine, 38*(5), 300–314.

Cohen, S., Doyle, W. J., & Skoner, D. P. (1999). Psychological stress, cytokine production, and severity of upper respiratory illness. *Psychosomatic Medicine, 61*(2), 175–180.

Corter, A. L., & Petrie, K. J. (2008). Expressive writing in context: The effects of a confessional setting and delivery of instructions on participant experience and language in writing. *British Journal of Health Psychology, 13*(1), 27–30.

Craft, M. A., Davis, G. C., & Paulson, R. M. (2012). Expressive writing in early breast cancer survivors. *Journal of Advanced Nursing, 69*(2), 305–315.

Creswell, D. J., Way, B. M., Eisenberger, N. I., & Lieberman, M. D. (2007). Neural correlates of dispositional mindfulness during affect labeling. *Psychosomatic Medicine, 69*(6), 560–565.

Cummings, J. A., Hayes, A. M., Saint, D. S., & Park, J. (2014). Expressive writing in psychotherapy: A tool to promote and track therapeutic change. *Professional Psychology: Research and Practice, 45,* 378–386.

Danoff-Burg, S., Agee, J. D., Romanoff, N. R., Kremer, J. M., & Strosberg, J. M. (2006). Benefit finding and expressive writing in adults with lupus or rheumatoid arthritis. *Psychology and Health, 21*(5), 651–665.

de Moor, C., Sterner, J., Hall, M., Warneke, C., Gilani, Z., Amato, R., et al. (2002). A pilot study of the effects of expressive writing on psychological and behavioral adjustment in patients enrolled in a Phase II trial of vaccine therapy for metastatic renal cell carcinoma. *Health Psychology, 21*(6), 615–619.

Dere-Meyer, C., Bender, B., Metzl, E., & Diaz, K. (2011). Psychotropic medication and art therapy: Overview of literature and clinical considerations. *The Arts in Psychotherapy, 38*(1), 29–35.

Deters, P. B., & Range, L. M. (2003). Does writing reduce posttraumatic stress disorder symptoms? *Violence and Victims, 18,* 569–580.

Dolev-Cohen, M., & Barak, A. (2013). Adolescents' use of instant messaging as a means of emotional relief. *Computers in Human Behavior, 29,* 58–63.

Dominguez, B., Valderrama, P., Meza, M. A., Perez, S. L., Silva, A., Martinez, G., et al. (1995). The roles of emotional reversal and disclosure in clinical practice. In J. W. Pennebaker (Ed.), *Emotion, Disclosure, and Health* (pp. 255–270). Washington, DC: American Psychological Association.

Donnelly, D. A., & Murray, E. J. (1991). Cognitive and emotional changes in written essays and therapy interviews. *Journal of Social and Clinical Psychology, 10,* 334–350.

Drake, J. E., & Winner, E. (2012). Confronting sadness through art-making: Distraction is more beneficial than venting. *Psychology of Aesthetics, Creativity, and the Arts, 6*(3), 255–261.

East, P., Startup, H., Roberts, C., & Schmidt, U. (2010). Expressive writing and eating disorder features: A preliminary trial in a student sample of the impact of three writing tasks on eating disorder symptoms and associated cognitive, affective and interpersonal factors. *European Eating Disorders Review, 18,* 180–196.

Einstein, G. O., Morris, J., & Smith, S. (1985). Note-taking, individual differences, and memory for lecture information. *Journal of Educational Psychology, 77*(5), 522–532.

Elbow, P. (1981). *Writing with Power.* New York: Oxford University Press.

Erickson, M. H., & Rossi, W. L. (1981). *Experiencing Hypnosis: Therapeutic Approaches to Altered States.* New York: Irvington.

Esterling, B. A., Antoni, M. H., Fletcher, M. A., Margulies, S., & Schneiderman, N. (1994). Emotional disclosure through writing or speaking modulates latent Epstein-Barr virus antibody titers. *Journal of Consulting and Clinical Psychology, 62*(1), 130–140.

Esterling, B. A., Antoni, M. H., Kumar, M., & Schneiderman, N. (1993). Defensiveness, trait anxiety, and Epstein-Barr viral capsid antigen antibody titers in healthy college students. *Health Psychology, 12*(2), 132–139.

Facchin, F., Margola, D., Molgora, S., & Revenson, T. A. (2014). Effects of benefit-focused versus standard expressive writing on adolescents' self-concept during the high school transition. *Journal of Research on Adolescence, 24*(1), 131–144.

Fisher, S. (1988). Leaving home: Homesickness and the psychological effects of change and transition. In S. Fisher & J. Reason (Eds.), *Handbook of Life Stress, Cognition and Health* (pp. 41–59). New York: Wiley.

Fowles, D. C. (1980). The three arousal model: Implications of Gray's two-factor learning theory for heart rate, electrodermal activity, and psychopathy. *Psychophysiology, 17*(2), 87–104.

Francis, M. E., & Pennebaker, J. W. (1992). Putting stress into words: Writing about personal upheavals and health. *American Journal of Health Promotion, 6*(1), 280–287.

Frankl, V. (1960). Paradoxical intention: A logotherapeutic technique. *American Journal of Psychotherapy, 14,* 520–525.

Frattaroli, J. (2006). Experimental disclosure and its moderators: A meta-analysis. *Psychological Bulletin, 132*(6), 823–865.

Frattaroli, J., Thomas, M., & Lyubomirsky, S. (2011). Opening up in the classroom: Effects of expressive writing on graduate school entrance exam performance. *Emotion, 11*(3), 691–696.

Freud, S. (1920/1966). *Introductory Lectures on Psychoanalysis*. New York: Norton.

Freud, S. (1961). *Civilization and Its Discontents*. London: Hogarth Press.

Freud, S. (1963). *Therapy and Technique*. New York: Collier.

Freud, S. (1965). *The Interpretation of Dreams*. New York: Avon.

Frisina, P. G., Borod, J. C., & Lepore, S. J. (2004). A meta-analysis of the effects of written emotional disclosure on the health outcomes of clinical populations. *Journal of Nervous and Mental Disease, 192*(9), 629–634.

Gersten, R., & Baker, S. (2001). Teaching expressive writing to students with learning disabilities: A meta-analysis. *Elementary School Journal, 101*(3), 251–272.

Gillis, M. E., Lumley, M. A., Mosley-Williams, A., Leisen, J. C. C., & Roehrs, T. (2006). The health effects of at-home written emotional disclosure in fibromyalgia: A randomized trial. *Annals of Behavioral Medicine, 32*(2), 135–146.

Glaser, R., & Kiecolt-Glaser, J. K. (1994). *Handbook of Human Stress and Immunity*. San Diego, CA: Academic Press.

Goleman, D. (1995). *Emotional Intelligence*. New York: Bantam.

Gordon, D. H., Baucom, D., & Snyder, K. C. (2007). An integrative intervention for promoting recovery from extramarital affairs. *Journal of Marital and Family Therapy, 30*(2), 213–231.

Gortner, E., Rude, S. S., & Pennebaker, J. W. (2006). Benefits of expressive writing in lowering rumination and depressive symptoms. *Behavior Therapy, 37*, 292–303.

Graf, M. C., Gaudiano, B. A., & Geller, P. A. (2008). Written emotional disclosure: A controlled study of the benefits of expressive writing homework in outpatient psychotherapy. *Psychotherapy Research, 18*, 389–399.

Graham, J., Lobel, M., Glass, P., & Lokshina, I. (2008). Effects of written anger expression in chronic pain patients: Making meaning from pain. *Journal of Behavioral Medicine, 31*, 201–212.

Graves, D., & Stuart, V. (1985). *Write from the Start: Tapping Your Child's Natural Writing Ability*. New York: New American Library.

Gray, J. (1975). *Elements of a Two-Factor Theory in Learning*. New York: Academic Press.

Greenberg, M. A., & Stone, A. A. (1992). Writing about disclosed versus undisclosed traumas: Immediate and long-term effects on mood and health. *Journal of Personality and Social Psychology, 63*, 75–84.

Greenberg, M. A., Wortman, C. B., & Stone, A. A. (1996). Emotional expression and physical health: Revising traumatic memories or fostering self-regulation. *Journal of Personality and Social Psychology, 71*(3), 588–602.

Hagen, A. M., Braasch, J. L. G., & Braten, I. (2014). Relationships between spontaneous notetaking, self-reported strategies and comprehension when reading multiple texts in different task conditions. *Journal of Research in Reading, 37*(S1), S141–S157.

Halpert, A., Rybin, D., & Doros, G. (2010). Expressive writing is a promising therapeutic modality for the management of IBS: A pilot study. *American Journal of Gastroenterology, 105*(11), 2440–2448.

Harris, A. H., 2006. Does expressive writing reduce health care utilization?: A meta analysis of randomized trials. *Journal of Consulting and Clinical Psychology 74,* 243–252.

Harvey, A. G., & Farrell, C. (2003). The efficacy of a Pennebaker-like writing intervention for poor sleepers. *Behavioral Sleep Medicine, 1*(2), 115–124.

Hevey, D., Wilczkiewicz, E., & Horgan, J. H. (2012). Type D moderates the effects of expressive writing on health-related quality of life (HRQOL) following myocardial infarction (MI). *Irish Journal of Psychology, 33*(2–3), 107–114.

Hirai, M., Skidmore, S. T., Clum, G. A., & Dolma, S. (2012). An investigation of the efficacy of online expressive writing for trauma-related psychological distress in Hispanic individuals. *Behavior Therapy, 43*(4), 812–824.

Holman, E. A., & Cohen Silver, R. (1998). Getting "stuck" in the past: Temporal orientation and coping with trauma. *Journal of Personality and Social Psychology, 74*(5), 1146–1163.

Horowitz, M. J. (1976). *Stress Response Syndromes.* New York: Jason Aronson.

Horowitz, M. J. (1987). *States of Mind.* New York: Plenum Press.

Hoyt, M. A., Austenfeld, J., & Stanton, A. L. (2014, September 29). Processing coping methods in expressive essays about stressful experiences: Predictors of health benefit. *Journal of Health Psychology.* E-publication ahead of print: pii: 1359105314550347.

Hsu, M. C., Schubiner, H., Lumley, M. A., Stracks, J. S., Clauw, D. J., & Williams, D. A. (2010). Sustained pain reduction through affective self-awareness in fibromyalgia: A randomized controlled trial. *Journal of General Internal Medicine, 25*(10), 1064–1070.

Ironson, G., O'Cleirigh, C., Leserman, J., Stuetzle, R., Fordiani, J., Fletcher, M., et al. (2013). Gender-specific effects of an augmented written emotional disclosure intervention on posttraumatic, depressive and HIV-disease-related outcomes: A randomized, controlled trial. *Journal of Consulting and Clinical Psychology, 81*(2), 284–298.

Janoff-Bulman, R. (1992). *Shattered Assumptions: Towards a New Psychology of Trauma.* New York: Free Press.

Jensen-Johansen, M. B., Christensen, S., Valdimarsdottir, H., Zakowski, S., Jensen, A. B., Bovbjerg, D. H., et al. (2013). Effects of an expressive writing intervention on cancer related distress in Danish breast cancer survivors—Results from a nationwide randomized clinical trial. *Psycho-Oncology, 22*(7), 1492–1500.

Junghaenel, D. U., Schwartz, J. E., & Broderick, J. E. (2008). Differential efficacy of written emotional disclosure for subgroups of fibromyalgia patients. *British Journal of Health Psychology, 13,* 57–60.

Junghaenel, D. U., Smyth, J. M., & Santner, L. (2008). Linguistic dimensions of psychopathology: A quantitative analysis. *Journal of Social and Clinical Psychology, 27*(1), 36–55.

Juth, V., Smyth, J., Carey, M., & Lepore, S. (2015). Social constraints are associated with negative psychological and physical adjustment in bereavement. *Applied Psychology: Health and Well-Being, 7*(2), 129–148.

Kabat-Zinn, J. (2003). Mindfulness-based interventions in context: Past, present, and future. *Clinical Psychology, 10*, 144–156.

Kagan, J., Reznick, S., & Snidman, N. (1988). Biological bases of childhood shyness. *Science, 240*, 167–171.

Kagan, J., Snidman, N., Julia-Sellers, M., & Johnson, M. O. (1991). Temperament and allergic symptoms. *Psychosomatic Medicine, 53*(3), 332–340.

Kalantari, M., Yule, W., Dyregrov, A., Neshatdoost, H., & Ahmadi, S. J. (2012). Efficacy of writing for recovery on traumatic grief symptoms of Afghani refugee bereaved adolescents: A randomized control trial. *OMEGA—Journal of Death and Dying, 65*(2), 139–150.

Kelly, A. E., & McKillop, K. J. (1996). Consequences of revealing personal secrets. *Psychological Bulletin, 120*, 450–465.

Kidd, D. C., & Castano, E. (2013). Reading literary fiction improves theory of mind. *Science, 342*, 377–380.

Kiepe, M. S., Stöckigt, B., & Keil, T. (2012). Effects of dance therapy and ballroom dances on physical and mental illnesses: A systematic review. *The Arts in Psychotherapy, 39*(5), 404–411.

Kircanski, K., Lieberman, M. D., & Craske, M. G. (2012). Feelings into words: Contributions of language to exposure therapy. *Psychological Science, 23*, 1086–1091.

Kirk, B. A., Schutte, N. S., & Hine, D. W. (2011). The effect of an expressive-writing intervention for employees on emotional self-efficacy, emotional intelligence, affect, and workplace incivility. *Journal of Applied Social Psychology, 41*(1), 179–195.

Klein, K., & Boals, A. (2001a). The relationship of life event stress and working memory capacity. *Applied Cognitive Psychology, 15*(5), 565–579.

Klein, K., & Boals, A. (2001b). Expressive writing can increase working memory capacity. *Journal of Experimental Psychology: General, 130*(3), 520.

Koopman, C., Ismailji, T., Holmes, D., Classen, C. C., Palesh, O., & Wales, T. (2005). The effects of expressive writing on pain, depression, and post-traumatic stress disorder symptoms in survivors of intimate partner violence. *Journal of Health Psychology, 10*(2), 211–221.

Koschwanez, H. E., Kerse, N., Darragh, M., Jarrett, P., Booth, R. J., & Broadbent, E. (2013). Expressive writing and wound healing in older adults: A randomized controlled trial. *Psychosomatic Medicine, 75*(6), 581–590.

Kovac, S. H., & Range, L. M. (2000). Writing projects: Lessening undergraduates' unique suicidal bereavement. *Suicide and Life-Threatening Behavior, 30*, 50–60.

Krantz, A. M., & Pennebaker, J. W. (2007). Expressive dance, writing, trauma, and health: When words have a body. In I. A. Serlin, J. Sonke-Henderson, R. Brandman, & J. Graham-Pole (Eds.), *Whole Person Healthcare: Vol. 3. The Arts and Health* (pp. 201–229). Westport, CT: Praeger.

Kross, E., & Ayduk, O. (2011). Making meaning out of negative experiences by self-distancing. *Current Directions in Psychological Science, 20*(3), 187–191.

Kross, E., Verduyn, P., Demiral, E., Park, J., Seungjae, L., Lin, N., et al. (2013). Facebook use predicts declines in subjective well-being in young adults. *PLoS ONE, 8,* e69841.

Krpan, K. M., Kross, E., Berman, M. G., Deldin, P. J., Askren, M. K., & Jonides, J. (2013). An everyday activity as a treatment for depression: The benefits of expressive writing for people diagnosed with major depressive disorder. *Journal of Affective Disorders, 150*(3), 1148–1151.

Kübler-Ross, E. (1966). *On Death and Dying*. Toronto: Macmillan.

Lange, A., Rietdijk, D., Hudcovicova, M., Van de Ven, J. P., Schrieken, B., & Emmelkamp, P. M. G. (2003). Interapy: A controlled randomized trial of the standardized treatment of posttraumatic stress through the Internet. *Journal of Consulting and Clinical Psychology, 71*(5), 901–909.

Lange, A., Van De Ven, J. Q., Schrieken, B. A. L., Bredeweg, B., & Emmelkamp, P. M. G. (2000). Internet-mediated, protocol-driven treatment of psychological dysfunction. *Journal of Telemedicine and Telecare, 6*(1), 15–21.

Langer, E. J. (1989). *Mindlessness*. Reading, MA: Addison-Wesley.

Leary, M. R. (1995). *Self-presentation: Impression Management and Interpersonal Behavior*. Madison, WI: Brown & Benchmark.

Leary, M. R., Tate, E. B., Adams, C. E., Batts Allen, A., & Hancock, J. (2007). Self-compassion and reactions to unpleasant self-relevant events: The implications of treating oneself kindly. *Journal of Personality and Social Psychology, 92*(5), 887–904.

Lepore, S. (1997). Expressive writing moderates the relation between intrusive thoughts and depressive symptoms. *Journal of Personality and Social Psychology, 73*(5), 1030–1037.

Lepore, S. J. (2001). A social–cognitive processing model of emotional adjustment to cancer. In A. L. Baum & B. L. Anderson (Eds.), *Psychosocial Interventions for Cancer* (pp. 94–116). Washington, DC: American Psychological Association.

Lepore, S. J., Fernandez-Berrocal, P., Ragan, J., & Ramos, N. (2004). It's not that bad: Social challenges to emotional disclosure enhance adjustment to stress. *Anxiety, Stress and Coping, 17*(4), 341–361.

Lepore, S. J., & Greenberg, M. A. (2002). Mending broken hearts: Effects of expressive writing on mood, cognitive processing, social adjustment and health following a relationship breakup. *Psychology and Health, 17*(5), 547–560.

Lewin, K. (1935). *A Dynamic Theory of Personality*. New York: McGraw-Hill.

Lewis, R. J., Derlega, V. J., Clarke, E. G., Kuang, J. L., Jacobs, A. M., & McElligott, M. D. (2005). An expressive writing intervention to cope with lesbian-related stress: The moderating effects of openness about sexual orientation. *Psychology of Women Quarterly, 29*(2), 149–157.

Lichtenthal, W. G., & Cruess, D. G. (2010). Effects of directed written disclosure on grief and distress symptoms among bereaved individuals. *Death Studies, 34*(6), 475–499.

Lumley, M. A., Keefe, F. J., Mosley-Williams, A., Rice, J. R., McKee, D., Waters, S. J., et al. (2014). The effects of written emotional disclosure and coping skills training in rheumatoid arthritis: A randomized clinical trial. *Journal of Consulting and Clinical Psychology, 82*(4), 644–658.

Lumley, M. A., Leegstra, S., Provenzano, K., & Warren, V. (1999). The health effects of writing about emotional stress on physically symptomatic young adults. *Psychosomatic Medicine, 61,* 89.

Lumley, M. A., Leisen, J. C. C., Partridge, R. T., Meyer, T. M., Radcliffe, A. M., Macklem, D. J., et al. (2011). Does emotional disclosure about stress improve health in rheumatoid arthritis?: Randomized controlled trials of written and spoken disclosure. *Pain, 152,* 866–877.

Lumley, M. A., & Provenzano, K. M. (2003). Stress management through written emotional disclosure improves academic performance among college students with physical symptoms. *Journal of Educational Psychology, 95*(3), 641–649.

Luria, A. R. (1981). *Language and Cognition.* New York: Wiley.

Makenzie, C. S., Wiprzycka, U. J., Hasher, L., & Goldstein, D. (2008). Seeing the class half full: Optimistic expressive writing improves mental health among chronically stressed caregivers. *British Journal of Health Psychology, 13,* 73–76.

Mann, T. (2001). Effects of future writing and optimism on health behaviors in HIV-infected women. *Annals of Behavioral Medicine, 23*(1), 26–33.

Marrington, C., & Troop, N. (2014). *A Study Exploring the Use of Expressive Writing to Reduce Stress in Parents of Children with Autism Spectrum Disorders.* Poster session presented at the annual conference of the British Psychological Society, Birmingham, UK.

Maslach, C. (1982). *Burnout: The Cost of Caring.* New York: Prentice Hall.

Maslow, A. (1968). *Toward a Psychology of Being* (2nd ed.). Princeton, NJ: Van Nostrand Reinhold.

McGuire, K. M. B., Greenberg, M. A., & Gevirtz, R. (2005). Autonomic effects of expressive writing in individuals with elevated blood pressure. *Journal of Health Psychology, 10*(2), 197–209.

Meij, L., Stroebe, M., Schut, H., Stroebe, W., Bout, J., Heijden, P., et al. (2008). Parents grieving the loss of their child: Interdependence in coping. *British Journal of Clinical Psychology, 47*(1), 31–42.

Merz, E. L., Fox, R. S., & Malcarne, V. L. (2014). Expressive writing interventions in cancer patients: A systematic review. *Health Psychology Review, 8*(3), 339–361.

Meshberg-Cohen, S., Svikis, D., & McMahon, T. J. (2014). Expressive writing as a therapeutic process for drug dependent women. *Substance Abuse, 35*(1), 80–88.

Mitchell, J. T., & Everly, G. S. (1995). Critical incident stress debriefing (CISD) and the prevention of work-related traumatic stress among high risk occupational groups. In G. S. Everly & J. M. Lating (Eds.), *Psychotraumatology: Key Papers and Core Concepts in Posttraumatic Stress* (pp. 267–280). New York: Plenum Press.

Mooney, P., Espie, C. A., & Broomfield, N. M. (2009). An experimental assessment of a Pennebaker writing intervention in primary insomnia. *Behavioral Sleep Medicine, 7*(2), 99–105.

Moore, S. D., Brody, L. R., & Dierberger, A. E. (2009). Mindfulness and experiential avoidance as predictors and outcomes of the narrative emotional disclosure task. *Journal of Clinical Psychology, 65*(9), 971–988.

Mosher, C. E., DuHamel, K. N., Lam, J., Dickler, M., Li, Y., Massie, M. J., et al. (2012). Randomised trial of expressive writing for distressed metastatic breast cancer patients. *Psychology and Health, 27*(1), 88–100.

Murray, E. J., Lamnin, A. D., & Carver, C. S. (1989). Emotional expression in written essays and psychotherapy. *Journal of Social and Clinical Psychology, 8*(4), 414–429.

Nazarian, D., & Smyth, J. M. (2010). Context moderates the effect of an expressive writing intervention: A randomized two-study replication and extension. *Journal of Social and Clinical Psychology, 29*(8), 903–929.

Nazarian, D., & Smyth, J. M. (2013). An experimental test of instructional manipulations in expressive writing interventions: Examining processes of change. *Journal of Social and Clinical Psychology, 32*(1), 71–96.

Neff, K. (2003). Self-compassion: An alternative conceptualization of a healthy attitude toward oneself. *Self and Identity, 2*(2), 85–101.

Nolen-Hoeksema, S. (1990). *Sex Differences in Depression.* Stanford, CA: Stanford University Press.

Nolen-Hoeksema, S., Parker, L. E., & Larson, J. (1994). Ruminative coping with depressed mood following loss. *Journal of Personality and Social Psychology, 67,* 92–104.

O'Cleirigh, C., Ironson, G., Antoni, M., Fletcher, M., McGuffey, L., Balbin, E., et al. (2003). Emotional expression and depth processing of trauma and their relation to long-term survival in patients with HIV/AIDS. *Journal of Psychosomatic Research, 54*(3), 225–235.

O'Connor, D. B., Hurling, R., Hendrickx, H., Osborne, G., Hall, J., Walklet, E., et al. (2011). Effects of written emotional disclosure on implicit self-esteem and body image. *British Journal of Health Psychology, 16*(3), 488–501.

Pachankis, J. E., & Goldfried, M. R. (2010). Expressive writing for gay-related stress: Psychosocial benefits and mechanisms underlying improvement. *Journal of Consulting and Clinical Psychology, 78,* 98–110.

Park, C. L. (2010). Making sense of the meaning literature: An integrative review of meaning making and its effects on adjustment to stressful life events. *Psychological Bulletin, 136*(2), 257–301.

Parkes, C. (2008). *Love and Loss: The Roots of Grief and Its Complications.* New York: Routledge.

Paudyal, P., Hine, P., Theadom, A., Apfelbacher, C. J., Jones, C. J., Yorke, J., et al. (2014, May 19). Written emotional disclosure for asthma review. *Cochrane Database of Systematic Reviews,* Issue 5.

Pennebaker, J. W. (1982). *The Psychology of Physical Symptoms.* New York: Springer-Verlag.

Pennebaker, J. W. (1989). Confession, inhibition, and disease. In L. Berkowitz (Ed.), *Advances in Experimental Social Psychology* (Vol. 22, pp. 211–244). New York: Academic Press.

Pennebaker, J. W. (1991). Self-expressive writing: Implications for health, education, and welfare. In S. I. Fontaine, P. Elbow, & P. Belanoff (Eds.), *Nothing Begins with N: New Investigations of Freewriting* (pp. 157–172). Carbondale: Southern Illinois Press.

Pennebaker, J. W. (1993). Putting stress into words: Health, linguistic, and therapeutic implications. *Behaviour Research and Therapy, 31*, 539–548.

Pennebaker, J. W. (Ed.). (1995). *Emotion, Disclosure, and Health*. Washington, DC: American Psychological Association.

Pennebaker, J. W. (2004). Theories, therapies, and taxpayers: On the complexities of the expressive writing paradigm. *Clinical Psychology: Science and Practice, 11*(2), 138–142.

Pennebaker, J. W. (2010). Expressive writing in a clinical setting. *Independent Practitioner, 30*(Winter), 23–25.

Pennebaker, J. W. (2011). *The Secret Life of Pronouns: What Our Words Say about Us*. New York: Bloomsbury.

Pennebaker, J. W., Barger, S. D., & Tiebout, J. (1989). Disclosure of traumas and health among Holocaust survivors. *Psychosomatic Medicine, 51*, 577–589.

Pennebaker, J. W., & Beall, S. K. (1986). Confronting a traumatic event: Toward an understanding of inhibition and disease. *Journal of Abnormal Psychology, 95*, 274–281.

Pennebaker, J. W., Booth, R. J., Boyd, R. L., & Francis, M. E. (2015). *Linguistic Inquiry and Word Count: LIWC2015*. Austin, TX: Pennebaker Conglomerates. (*www.LIWC.net*)

Pennebaker, J. W., & Chew, C. H. (1985). Behavioral inhibition and electrodermal activity during deception. *Journal of Personality and Social Psychology, 49*, 1427–1433.

Pennebaker, J. W., & Chung, C. K. (2011). Expressive writing and its links to mental and physical health. In H. S. Friedman (Ed.), *Oxford Handbook of Health Psychology* (pp. 417–437). New York: Oxford University Press.

Pennebaker, J. W., Colder, M., & Sharp, L. K. (1990). Accelerating the coping process. *Journal of Personality and Social Psychology, 58*, 528–537.

Pennebaker, J. W., Czajka, J. A., Cropanzano, R., Richards, B. C., in collaboration with Brumbelow, S., Ferrara, K., et al. (1990). Levels of thinking. *Personality and Social Psychology Bulletin, 16*, 743–757.

Pennebaker, J. W., & Evans, J. F. (2014). *Expressive Writing: Words That Heal*. Enumclaw, WA: Idyll Arbor.

Pennebaker, J. W., & Francis, M. E. (1996). Cognitive, emotional, and language processes in disclosure. *Cognition and Emotion, 10*, 601–626.

Pennebaker, J. W., Francis, M. E., & Booth, R. J. (2001). *Linguistic Inquiry and Word Count: LIWC2001*. Mahwah, NJ: Erlbaum.

Pennebaker, J. W., Hughes, C. F., & O'Heeron, R. C. (1987). The psychophysiology of confession: Linking inhibitory and psychosomatic processes. *Journal of Personality and Social Psychology, 52*, 781–793.

Pennebaker, J. W., Kiecolt-Glaser, J., & Glaser, R. (1988). Disclosure of traumas and immune function: Health implications for psychotherapy. *Journal of Consulting and Clinical Psychology, 56*, 239–245.

Pennebaker, J. W., & King, L. (1999). Linguistic style: Language use as an individual difference. *Journal of Personality and Social Psychology, 77*, 1296–1312.

Pennebaker, J. W., Mayne, T. J., & Francis, M. E. (1997). Linguistic predictors of adaptive bereavement. *Journal of Personality and Social Psychology, 72*(4), 863–871.

Pennebaker, J. W., & O'Heeron, R. C. (1984). Confiding in others and illness rates among spouses of suicide and accidental death. *Journal of Abnormal Psychology, 93*, 473–476.

Pennebaker, J. W., & Susman, J. R. (1988). Disclosure of traumas and psychosomatic processes. *Social Science and Medicine, 26*, 327–332.

Pennebaker, J. W., & Traue, H. C. (1993). Inhibition and psychosomatic processes. In H. C. Traue & J. W. Pennebaker (Eds.), *Emotion, Inhibition, and Health* (pp. 146–163). Seattle, WA: Hogrefe & Huber.

Petrie, K. J., Booth, R., Pennebaker, J. W., Davison, K. P., & Thomas, M. (1995). Disclosure of trauma and immune response to Hepatitis B vaccination program. *Journal of Consulting and Clinical Psychology, 63*(5), 787–792.

Petrie, K. J., Fontanilla, I., Thomas, M. G., Booth, R. J., & Pennebaker, J. W. (2004). Effect of written emotional expression on immune function in patients with human immunodeficiency virus infection: A randomized trial. *Psychosomatic Medicine, 66*, 272–275.

Range, L. M., & Jenkins, S. R. (2010). Who benefits from Pennebaker's expressive writing paradigm?: Research recommendations from three gender theories. *Sex Roles, 63*, 149–164.

Range, L. M., Kovac, S. H., & Marion, M. S. (2000). Does writing about the bereavement lessen grief following sudden, unintentional death? *Death Studies, 24*, 115–134.

Richards, J. M., Beal, W. E., Seagal, J., & Pennebaker, J. W. (2000). The effects of disclosure of traumatic events on illness behavior among psychiatric prison inmates. *Journal of Abnormal Psychology, 109*, 156–160.

Rimé, B. (1995). Mental rumination, social sharing, and the recovery from emotional exposure. In J. W. Pennebaker (Ed.), *Emotion, Disclosure, and Health* (pp. 271–291). Washington, DC: American Psychological Association.

Rogers, C. (1951). *Client-Centered Therapy.* Boston: Houghton-Mifflin.

Rosenberg, H. J., Rosenberg, S. D., Ernstoff, M. S., Wolford, G. L., Amdur, R. J., Elshamy, M. R., et al. (2002). Expressive disclosure and health outcomes in a prostate cancer population. *International Journal of Psychiatry in Medicine, 32*, 37–53.

Rubenstein, C. (1982). Wellness is all: A report on *Psychology Today*'s survey of beliefs about health. *Psychology Today, 16*, 28–37.

Salloum, A., & Overstreet, S. (2012). Grief and trauma intervention for children after disaster: Exploring coping skills versus trauma narration. *Behaviour Research and Therapy, 50*(3), 169–179.

Sapolsky, R. M. (1994). *Why Zebras Don't Get Ulcers*. New York: Freeman.

Schilte, A. F., Portegijs, P. J. M., Blankenstein, A. H., van der Horst, H. E., Latour, M. B. F., van Eijk, J. T. M., & Knottnerus, J. A. (2001). Randomised controlled trial of disclosure of emotionally important events in somatisation in primary care. *British Medical Journal, 323*, 86.

Schmidt, U., Bone, G., Hems, S., Lessem, J., & Treasure, J. (2002). Structured therapeutic writing tasks as an adjunct to treatment in eating disorders. *European Eating Disorders Review, 10*(5), 299–315.

Schooler, J. W., & Engstler-Schooler, T. Y. (1990). Verbal overshadowing of visual memories: Some things are better left unsaid. *Cognitive Psychology, 22*, 36–71.

Schwartz, G. E., & Kline, J. (1995). Repression, emotional disclosure, and health: Theoretical, empirical, and clinical considerations. In J. W. Pennebaker (Ed.), *Emotion, Disclosure, and Health* (pp. 177–194). Washington, DC: American Psychological Association.

Segal, D. L., & Murray, E. J. (1994). Emotional processing in cognitive therapy and vocal expression of feeling. *Journal of Social and Clinical Psychology, 13*, 189–206.

Seih, Y., Chung, C. K., & Pennebaker, J. W. (2011). Experimental manipulations of perspective taking and perspective switching in expressive writing. *Cognition and Emotion, 25*, 926–938.

Selman, L. E., Williams, J., & Simms, V. (2012). A mixed-methods evaluation of complementary therapy services in palliative care: Yoga and dance therapy. *European Journal of Cancer Care, 21*(1), 87–97.

Sheese, B. E., Brown, E. L., & Graziano, W. G. (2004). Emotional expression in cyberspace: Searching for moderators of the Pennebaker disclosure effect via e-mail. *Health Psychology, 23*, 457–464.

Shortt, J. W., & Pennebaker, J. W. (1992). Talking versus hearing about Holocaust experiences. *Basic and Applied Social Psychology, 13*, 165–179.

Silver, R. C., Boon, C., & Stones, M. H. (1983). Searching for meaning in misfortune: Making sense of incest. *Journal of Social Issues, 39*, 81–102.

Simmel, G. (1950). *The Sociology of Georg Simmel*. New York: Free Press.

Slatcher, R. B., & Pennebaker, J. W. (2006). How do I love thee? Let me count the words: The social effects of expressive writing. *Psychological Science, 17*(8), 660–664.

Sloan, D. M., Lee, D. J., Litwack, S. D., Sawyer, A. T., & Marx, B. P. (2013). Written exposure therapy for veterans diagnosed with PTSD: A pilot study. *Journal of Traumatic Stress, 26*(6), 776–779.

Sloan, D. M., Marx, B. P., Bovin, M. J., Feinstein, B. A., & Gallagher, M. W. (2012). Written exposure as an intervention for PTSD: A randomized clinical trial with motor vehicle accident survivors. *Behaviour Research and Therapy, 50*(10), 627–635.

Sloan, D. M., Marx, B. P., Epstein, E., & Dobbs, J. (2008). Expressive writing buffers against maladaptive rumination. *Emotion, 8*(2), 302–306.

Sloan, D. M., Marx, B. P., Epstein, E. M., & Lexington, J. M. (2007). Does altering the writing instructions influence outcome associated with written disclosure? *Behavior Therapy, 38*, 155–168.

Sloan, D. M., Marx, B. P., & Greenberg, E. M. (2011). A test of written emotional disclosure as an intervention for posttraumatic stress disorder.
Behaviour Research and Therapy, 49(4), 299–304.

Smith, H. E., Jones, C. J., Hankins, M., Field, A., Theadom, A., Bowskill, R.,
Horne, R., & Frew, A. J. (2015). The effects of expressive writing on lung
function, quality of life, medication use, and symptoms in adults with
asthma: A randomized controlled trial. *Psychosomatic Medicine, 77*(4),
429–437.

Smyth, J. M. (1998). Written emotional expression: Effect sizes, outcome
types, and moderating variables. *Journal of Consulting and Clinical Psychology, 66*(1), 174–184.

Smyth, J. M., & Helm, R. (2003). Focused expressive writing as self-help for
stress and trauma. *Journal of Clinical Psychology, 59*(2), 227–235.

Smyth, J. M., Hockemeyer, J. R., Heron, K., Wonderlich, S., & Pennebaker, J.
(2008). Prevalence, type, disclosure, and severity of trauma and adverse
events in college students. *Journal of American College Health, 57*, 69–76.

Smyth, J. M., Hockemeyer, J. R., & Tulloch, H. (2008). Expressive writing
and post-traumatic stress disorder: Effects on trauma symptoms, mood
states and cortisol reactivity. *British Journal of Health Psychology, 13*, 85–93.

Smyth, J. M., Nazarian, D., & Arigo, D. (2008). Expressive writing in the
clinical context. In J. Denollet, I. Nyklicek, & A. Vingerhoets (Eds.),
Emotion Regulation: Conceptual and Clinical Issues (pp. 215–233). New York:
Springer.

Smyth, J. M., & Pennebaker, J. W. (2008). Exploring the boundary conditions of expressive writing: In search of the right recipe. *British Journal of
Health Psychology, 13*, 1–7.

Smyth, J. M., Stone, A. A., Hurewitz, A., & Kaell, A. (1999). Effects of writing about stressful experiences on symptom reduction in patients with
asthma or rheumatoid arthritis. *Journal of the American Medical Association, 281*(14), 1304–1309.

Smyth, J. M., True, N., & Souto, J. (2001). Effects of writing about traumatic
experiences: The necessity for narrative structure. *Journal of Social and
Clinical Psychology, 20*, 161–172.

Snyder, D. K., Gordon, K. C., & Baucom, D. H. (2004). Treating affair couples:
Extending the written disclosure paradigm to relationship trauma. *Clinical Psychology: Science and Practice, 11*(2), 155–159.

Spera, S. P., Buhrfeind, E. D., & Pennebaker, J. W. (1994). Expressive writing
and coping with job loss. *Academy of Management Journal, 37*, 722–733.

Stanton, A. L., Danoff-Burg, S., Sworowski, L. A., Collins, C. A., Branstetter,
A. D., Rodriguez Hanley, A., et al. (2002). Randomized controlled trial
of written emotional expression and benefit finding in breast cancer
patients. *Journal of Clinical Oncology, 20*, 4160–4168.

Stockton, H., Joseph, S., & Hunt, N. (2014). Expressive writing and posttraumatic growth: An Internet-based study. *Traumatology: An International
Journal, 20*(2), 75–83.

Stroebe, M., Finkenauer, C., Wijngaards-de Meij, L., Schut, H., van den Bout,
J., & Stroebe, W. (2013). Partner-oriented self-regulation among bereaved

parents: The costs of holding in grief for the partner's sake. *Psychological Science, 24*(4), 395–402.

Stroebe, M., Schut, H., & Stroebe, W. (2006). Who benefits from disclosure?: Exploration of attachment style differences in the effects of expressive emotions. *Clinical Psychology Review, 26,* 66–85.

Stroebe, M., Schut, H., & Stroebe, W. (2007). Health outcomes of bereavement. *Lancet, 370*(9603), 1960–1973.

Stroebe, M., Stroebe, W., & Hansson, R. O. (Eds.). (1993). *Handbook of Bereavement.* New York: Cambridge University Press.

Stroebe, M., Stroebe, W., Schut, H., Zech, E., & van den Bout, J. (2002). Does disclosure of emotions facilitate recovery from bereavement?: Evidence from two prospective studies. *Journal of Consulting and Clinical Psychology, 70*(1), 169–178.

Stuckey, H. L., & Nobel, J. (2010). The connection between art, healing, and public health: A review of current literature. *American Journal of Public Health, 100*(2), 254.

Swann, W. B. (1996). *Self-Traps: The Elusive Quest for Higher Self-Esteem.* New York: Freeman.

Taylor, S. E. (2014). *Health Psychology* (9th ed.). New York: McGraw-Hill.

Van Middendorp, H., Geenen, R., Sorbi, M. J., Van Doornen, L. J. P., & Bijlsma, J. W. J. (2009). Health and physiological effects of an emotional disclosure intervention adapted for application at home: A randomized clinical trial in rheumatoid arthritis. *Psychotherapy and Psychosomatics, 78*(3), 145–151.

Vygotsky, L. S. (1978). *Mind in Society* (M. Cole & colleagues, Eds.). Cambridge, MA: Harvard University Press.

Vygotsky, L. S. (1986). *Thought and Language* (A. Kozulin, Ed.). Cambridge, MA: MIT Press.

Wagner, L., Hilker, K., Hepworth, J., & Wallston, K. (2010). Cognitive adaptability as a moderator of expressive writing effects in an HIV sample. *AIDS and Behavior, 14*(2), 410–420.

Walker, B., Nail, L., & Croyle, R. (1999). Does emotional expression make a difference in reactions to breast cancer? *Oncology Nursing Forum, 26*(6), 1025–1032.

Walker, B., Shippen, M. E., Alberto, P., Houchins, D. E., & Cihak, D. F. (2006). Using the expressive writing program to improve the writing skills of high school students with learning disabilities. *Journal of Direct Instruction, 6*(1), 35–47.

Warner, L. J., Lumley, M. A., Casey, R. J., Pierantoni, W., Salazar, R., Zoratti, E. M., et al. (2006). Health effects of written emotional disclosure in adolescents with asthma: A randomized controlled trial. *Journal of Pediatric Psychology, 31*(6), 557–568.

Wegner, D. (1989). *White Bears and Other Unwanted Thoughts* (2nd ed.). New York: Guilford Press.

Wegner, D. M., Giuliano, T., & Hertel, P. T. (1985). Cognitive interdependence in close relationships. In W. Ickes (Ed.), *Compatible and Incompatible Relationships* (pp. 253–276). New York: Springer-Verlag.

Weinman, J., Ebrecht, M., Scott, S., Walburn, J., & Dyson, M. (2008). Enhanced wound healing after emotional disclosure intervention. *British Journal of Health Psychology, 13*, 95–102.

Wenzlaff, R. M., & Wegner, D. M. (2000). Thought suppression. *Annual Review of Psychology, 51*, 59–91.

Wetherell, M. A., Byrne-Davis, L., Dieppe, P., Donovan, J., Brookes, S., Byron, M., et al. (2005). Effects of emotional disclosure on psychological and physiological outcomes in patients with rheumatoid arthritis: An exploratory home-based study. *Journal of Health Psychology, 10*(2), 277–285.

Willmott, L., Harris, P., Gellaitry, G., Cooper, V., & Horne, R. (2011). The effects of expressive writing following first myocardial infarction: A randomized controlled trial. *Health Psychology, 30*(5), 642–650.

Wolf, S., & Goodell, H. (1968). *Harold G. Wolff's Stress and Disease.* Springfield, IL: Charles C Thomas.

Wood, M. J., Molassiotis, A., & Payne, S. (2011). What research evidence is there for the use of art therapy in the management of symptoms in adults with cancer?: A systematic review. *Psycho-Oncology, 20*(2), 135–145.

Wortman, C. B., & Silver, R. C. (1989). The myths of coping with loss. *Journal of Consulting and Clinical Psychology, 57*, 349–357.

Yogo, M., & Fujihara, S. (2008). Working memory capacity can be improved by expressive writing: A randomized experiment in a Japanese sample. *British Journal of Health Psychology, 13*, 77–80.

Zakowski, S. G., Ramati, A., Morton, C., Flanigan, R., & Johnson, P. (2004). Written emotional disclosure buffers the effects of social constraints on distress among cancer patients. *Health Psychology, 23*(6), 555–563.

Zeigarnik, B. W. (1927). Uber das Behalten von erledigten und unerledigten Handlungen. *Psychologische Forschung, 9*, 1–85.

Zhu, S. H., Stretch, V., Balabanis, M., Rosbrook, B., Sadler, G., & Pierce, J. P. (1996). Telephone counseling for smoking cessation: Effects of single-session and multiple-session interventions. *Journal of Consulting and Clinical Psychology, 64*(1), 202–211.

Author Index

Ahmadi, S. J., 179n
Ailey, A., 148
Altman, I., 128
Ames, S. C., 161, 174n
Arbus, D., 148
Arigo, D., 178n
Aristotle, 11, 77
Ayduk, O., 142

Baikie, K. A., 176n
Baker, S., 68
Bangert-Drowns, R. L., 68
Barak, A., 76
Baucom, D., 173n
Baucom, D. H., 179n
Beal, W. E., 175n
Beall, S. K., 16, 171n
Bernard, M., 61, 173n
Bliese, P. D., 177n
Boals, A., 68, 86, 173n
Bonanno, G. A., 178n
Bond, M., 176n
Bowlby, J., 105
Braasch, J. L. G., 176n
Braten, I., 176n
Breslau, N., 177n
Breuer, J., 11, 28, 29
Broadbent, L., 47
Brody, L. R., 178n
Broomfield, N. M., 178n
Brown, B., 40, 124, 177n

Cabrera, O. A., 177n
Cameron, L. D., 144
Castro, C. A., 177n
Chaudoir, S. R., 116

Chiesa, A., 178n
Chilcoat, H. D., 177n
Clum, G. A., 176n
Cobain, K., 148
Cobb, S., 122
Cohen, S., 180n
Cooper, V., 172n
Corter, A. L., 164
Creswell, D. J., 91
Cummings, J. A., 173n, 174n

Danoff-Burg, S., 52
Davis, G. C., 177n
de Moor, C., 178n
Deters, P. B., 175n
Dierberger, A. E., 178n
Dobbs, J., 173n
Dolma, S., 176n
Doros, G., 176n
Drake, J. E., 149
Dyregrov, A., 179n
Dyson, M., 172n

Ebrecht, M., 172n
Einstein, G. O., 71
Elbow, P., 71
Epstein, E., 173n
Erickson, M. H., 33
Espie, C. A., 178n

Farrell, C., 178n
Fisher, J. D., 116
Fosse, B., 148
Fowles, D. C., 172n
Francis, M. E., 150
Frankl, V., 84

Frattaroli, J., 173n
Freud, S., 7, 11, 29, 44, 88, 127, 137, 144
Fujihara, S., 173n

Gaudiano, B. A., 173n
Geerligs, L., 176n
Gellaitry, G., 172n
Geller, P. A., 173n
Gersten, R., 68
Gillis, M. E., 175n
Glaser, R., 19, 20
Goldfried, M. R., 174n
Goleman, D., 172n
Gordon, D. H., 173n, 180n
Gordon, K. C., 179n
Gortner, E., 173n, 178n
Graf, M. C., 173n
Graham, J., 142
Graves, D., 71
Greenberg, E. M., 161
Greenberg, M. A., 179n

Hagen, A. M., 176n
Halpert, A., 176n
Harris, P., 172n, 175n
Harvey, A. G., 178n
Hawthorne, N., 48
Hepworth, J., 174n
Hevey, D., 57
Hilker, K., 174n
Hirai, M., 176n
Hoge, C. W., 177n
Holman, E. A., 180n
Horne, R., 57, 172n
Horowitz, M. J., 99
Hsu, M. C., 52
Hughes, C. F., 35

Ironson, G., 54
Jackson, C., 173n
Janoff-Bulman, R., 139
Jones, C., 173n
Jung, C., 77
Juth, V., 118

Kabat-Zinn, J., 90, 178n
Kalantari, M., 179n
Kessler, R. C., 177n
Kidd, D. C., 181n
Kiecolt-Glaser, J. K., 19, 20
King, L., 143, 161
Klein, K., 68, 86, 173n
Koschwanez, H. E., 172n
Kovac, S. H., 175n
Krantz, A. M., 148, 181n
Kross, E., 76, 142
Krpan, K. M., 59
Kübler-Ross, E., 98, 99

Lange, A., 176n
Langer, E. J., 90
Lao-Tzu, 77
Leary, M. R., 91
Leegstra, S., 175n
Leisen, J. C. C., 175n
Lepore, S. J., 121, 173n, 179n, 181n
Lewin, K., 136
Lewis, R. J., 174n
Lieberman, M. D., 39, 91, 172n
Lumley, M. A., 52, 173n, 175n
Luria, A. R., 70
Lyubomirsky, S., 173n

Mahler, G., 148
Mann, T., 54
Marion, M. S., 175n
Marx, B. P., 173n
Maslach, C., 130
Maslow, A., 148
McGuire, K. M. B., 38, 57
Merz, E. L., 56
Messer, S. C., 177n
Mitchell, J. T., 102
Mooney, P., 178n
Moore, S. D., 91, 178n
Mosher, C. E., 173n
Mosley-Williams, A., 175n

Nail, L., 161
Napoleon, B, 78
Nazarian, D., 162
Neff, K., 91
Neshatdoost, H., 179n
Nicholls, G., 144
Nightingale, F., 163
Nobel, J., 148

O'Cleirigh, C., 53
O'Heeron, R. C., 35
O'Neill, E., 148
Overstreet, S., 179n

Pachankis, J. E., 174n
Parkes, C., 179n
Pennebaker, J. W., x, 2, 4, 5, 11, 12, 13,
    14, 16, 18, 19, 20, 34, 35, 36, 39, 43,
    66, 75, 78, 81, 87, 89, 93, 101, 110,
    117, 124, 125, 129, 130, 146, 147,
    150, 152, 171n, 173n, 175n, 176n,
    180n, 181n
Pepys, S., 74
Petrie, K. J., 53, 164
Plath, S., 148
Provenzano, K., 173n, 175n

Range, L. M., 175n
Richards, J. M., 175n

Rimé, B., 128
Roehrs, T., 175n
Rogers, C., 125, 144
Rosenberg, H. J., 175n
Rubenstein, C., 14
Rude, S. S., 173n
Rybin, D., 176n

Salloum, A., 179n
Sapolsky, R. M., 171n
Schilte, A. F., 175n
Schooler, J. W., 145
Schut, H., 175n, 179n
Scott, S., 172n
Seagal, J., 175n
Selman, L. E., 181n
Serretti, A., 178n
Silver, R., 100, 112, 139
Simmel, G., 125
Simms, V., 181n
Skidmore, S. T., 176n
Slatcher, R. B., 121, 122
Sloan, D. M., 61, 173n
Smith, H., 51
Smyth, J. M., x, 2, 5, 6, 24, 25, 39, 43,
     47, 51, 52, 62, 75, 78, 89, 125, 129,
     147, 152, 153, 162, 173n, 174n, 178n,
     181n
Snyder, D. K., 179n
Snyder, K. C., 173n
Spera, S. P., 22
Spinoza, B, 77
Stanton, A. L., 175n
Stockton, H., 176n
Stone, A., 24

Stone, A. A., 24, 161
Strayed, C., 148
Stroebe, M., 104, 121, 175n, 179n
Stroebe, W., 104, 175n, 179n
Stuckey, H. L., 148
Swann, W. B., 123

Taylor, D. A., 128
Taylor, S. E., 171n
Thomas, M., 173n

Van den Bout, J., 175n
van Gogh, V., 148
Vygotsky, L. S., 69, 70

Wagner, L., 174n
Walburn, J., 172n
Walker, B., 172n
Wallston, K., 174n
Warren, V., 175n
Wegner, D., 84, 85, 147, 177n
Weinman, J., 47, 172n
Wenzlaff, R. M., 177n
Wilhelm, K., 176n
Williams, J., 181n
Willmott, L., 172n
Wolf, S., 6, 7
Wolff, H. G., 6, 7
Woolf, V., 78
Wortman, C. B., 100, 112, 161

Yule, W., 179n

Zech, E., 175n
Zeigarnik, B. W., 136

Subject Index

Note: *f* or *n* following a page number indicates a figure or a note.

Acceptance, 91, 98–99, 177*n*
Addiction, 89–90
Adjustment
    college transition, 110–112
    expressive writing and, x, 55, 63,
        159–163
    leaning and health outcomes and, 69
Alcohol use, 89–90
Anger
    complaining and overdisclosing and,
        78–79
    coping with trauma and, 97–99, 113
    disease and, 48
    self-compassion and, 91
    unwanted thoughts and, 95
Anonymity, 125–126, 131–134, 168
Anxiety
    coping with trauma and, 113–114
    disease and, 48
    expressive writing and, ix–x, 18
    learning and health outcomes and,
        69
    lie detection confession effect and,
        4–5
    psychological links to health and
        illness, 7–9
    rumination and, 83–84
    suppression of thoughts and, 84
    unwanted thoughts and, 92
Approaches to expressive writing,
    163. *See also* Expressive writing
    technique
Art, 148–150, 181*n*
Arthritis. *See* Rheumatoid arthritis
Assimilation stage of coping, 99, 107–
    109. *See also* Acceptance; Coping
Assimilation stage of emotion, 106–107

Asthma, 43, 51, 63. *See also* Chronic
    health problems; Inflammation
Attachment, 105–106
Attentional focus, 48, 72–73, 94, 151–152
Authenticity, 40
Autoimmune disorders, 50–54, 59. *See*
    also Chronic health problems
Avoidance, 87–90

Bargaining, 98–99
Being-confronted note-taking strategy,
    71–72
Benefit finding approach to expressive
    writing, 143–144, 163. *See also*
    Expressive writing technique
Bereavement
    coping with, 104–107
    health and, 179*n*
    loss of social support following a
        death and, 118–120
    overview, 178*n*–179*n*
    talking about and reacting to trauma
        and, 117–118
Best possible future self approach to
    expressive writing, 163. *See also*
    Expressive writing technique
Biological mechanisms, 46–47
Bipolar disorder, 61–62
Blog writing, 76
Blood pressure, 7, 37, 56–57
Brain functions, 38–39
Burnout, 130–131

Cancers, 54–56, 59, 63, 172*n*. *See also*
    Chronic health problems
Cardiovascular disease, 56–58, 59, 63. *See*
    also Chronic health problems

Caregiving roles, 160
Care-seeking behavior, 175n
Catharsis, 28–30
Cause–effect relationships, 7, 8–10
Chronic health problems. See also Health
    benefits; Physical health problems
    biology and psychology of expressive
        writing and, 46–50
    care-seeking behavior and, 175n
    expressive writing and, 42–43, 50–64
    nature of diseases, 44–46
    overview, 172n
    self-care and, 49–50
    stages of coping and, 98–99
    when to use or not use expressive
        writing techniques, 160–161
Cognitive processes, 94, 153–154
Cognitive processing approach to
    expressive writing, 163. See also
    Expressive writing technique
Cognitive words, 151. See also Language
    use and development
College transition, 110–112
Compassion for the self. See Self-
    compassion
Complaining, 78–79
Completion, 136–137
Completion stage of coping, 99. See also
    Acceptance; Coping
Compulsions, 7–8, 82–83. See also
    Thoughts, intrusive and unwanted
Computer-based writing, 75–76
Confession. See also Disclosure
    benefits of, 135
    body's response to, 34–35
    brain functions during, 38–39
    complaining and overdisclosing and,
        78–79
    context or ritual in, 164
    health and, 2–6, 11
    high disclosers versus low disclosers,
        35–38
    laboratory's role in, 40–41
    letting-go experience and, 30–33
    overview, 1–2, 10–12
    physiology of, 33–34
    sleep and, 93–94
    substitutes to writing, 169
    values and, 131–134
Confronting note-taking strategy, 71–72
Contradictions, 4
Conversations, 2–3, 30–33, 144–146
Coping. See also Trauma
    altering thinking styles to avoid stress
        and, 89–90
    bereavement and, 104–107
    college transition, 110–112
    history of, 98–100

loss of social support following a
    death and, 118–120
marital problems following a shared
    trauma, 120–121
natural sequence of, 97–98
overview, 96–97, 112–114
psychotherapy and, 101–103
resilience and, 100–101
social support and, 115–117, 122–129
speeding up or slowing down, 96–97,
    110
support from others and, 101–103
Counseling, 101–103
Creativity, 71–73
Crises, ongoing, 112–113, 159–161
Critical incident stress debriefing (CISD),
    102–103
Cultural factors, 165

Dancing, 148–150, 181n
Death, 104–107, 118–120. See also Loss
Debriefing, 102–103
Denial, 7–8, 98–99, 113
Depression
    benefit finding and, 143–144
    coping with trauma and, 98–99,
        113–114
    expressive writing and, ix–x, 58–60,
        173n
    rumination and, 83–84
    sleep and, 93–94
    suppression of thoughts and, 84
    unwanted thoughts and, 92
Developmental processes, 70. See also
    Language use and development
Diabetes, 56–58. See also Chronic health
    problems
Diary writing, ix, 73–75, 107–109
Disclosure. See also Confession; Secrets
    benefit finding and, 144
    benefits of, 27–30, 135
    brain functions during, 38–39
    care-seeking behavior and, 175n
    catharsis versus insight and, 28–29
    choosing a confidant, 124–129
    complaining and overdisclosing and,
        78–79
    context or ritual in, 164
    diary writing and, 74–75
    disclosure process model, 154–157
    high disclosers versus low disclosers,
        35–38
    illness and health and, 11
    letting-go experience and, 30–33
    loss of social support following a
        death and, 118–120
    overview, 172n, 181n–182n
    professional help and, 126–127

Disclosure (*cont.*)
  relationship distress and, 121–122
  self-expression and, 148–150
  sleep and, 93–94, 178*n*
  social support and, 115–117, 180*n*
  stress reduction and, 147
  substitutes to writing, 169
  talking about and reacting to trauma
    and, 117–118
  translating experiences into language,
    144–146
  values and, 131–134
  when its helpful versus not helpful,
    122–123
Disclosure process model, 154–157
Distraction, 103, 114
Drawing, 148–150
Dreams, 137. *See also* Sleep
Drug use, 89–90
Duration of expressive writing, 163–164,
  166–167. *See also* Expressive writing
  technique

*E*ducation, x, 66–68, 68–71. *See also*
  Learning
Emotions
  disease and, 47–48
  emotion regulation, 91
  following an expressive writing
    session, 169
  psychological links to health and
    illness, 8
  stages of grief and love and, 106–109
Employment, 22–23, 140–142
Exercise, 89–90
Exposure approach to expressive
  writing, 163. *See also* Expressive
  writing technique
Expression of self. *See* Self-expression
Expressive drawing, 149
Expressive writing technique. *See also*
  Writing
  approaches to, 163
  assumptions regarding, 158–159
  benefit finding and, 143–144
  biology and psychology of, 46–50
  brain functions during, 38–39
  chronic health problems and, 50–64
  disclosure process model and,
    154–157
  duration, frequency, and spacing of
    writing sessions, 163–164, 166–167
  effectiveness of, 165–166
  focus on traumatic or negative
    experiences and, 161–163
  illness prevention and, 15–16
  immune system and, 19–22

  improving learning and health
    outcomes with, 68–71
  learning and creativity and, 71–73
  letting-go experience and, 30–33
  meta-analysis on, 24–26
  mindfulness and, 91
  occupational factors and, 22–23
  origin of, 16–19
  overview, ix–xi, 26, 65–66, 158–159,
    166–170
  relationship distress and, 121–122
  role of narrative and, 152–153
  sleep and, 93–94, 178*n*
  summarizing and sharing memory
    and, 147
  as a tool for education, 66–68
  translating experiences into language,
    150–152
  understanding the unfathomable and,
    139–140
  values and, 131–134
  what to write about, 62–63
  when to use or not use, 159–161
  who may benefit from, 165–166

*F*acebook, 75–76
Fear, 40, 48
Fibromyalgia, 52
Focus, 48, 72–73, 94
Formal thinking, 69. *See also* Thinking
  abilities
Formal writing, 73. *See also* Writing
Freewriting, 19, 70–71, 73. *See also* Writing
Frequency of expressive writing, 163–
  164, 166–167. *See also* Expressive
  writing technique
Friendship. *See also* Social support
  choosing a confidant, 124–129
  disclosure and, 122–123, 128, 180*n*
  love and, 107
  secrets and, 180*n*
  support from others and, 101–103
  working memory and, 154
  writing as a replacement for, 80

*G*ender differences, 54, 74
Greed, 91
Grief. *See also* Bereavement; Loss; Trauma
  benefit finding and, 143–144
  example of, 107–109
  loss of social support following a
    death and, 118–120
  overview, 105, 113–114, 178*n*–179*n*
  speeding up or slowing down, 110
  stages of, 98–99, 106–109
  when to use or not use expressive
    writing techniques, 160

Habits, 44
Health benefits. *See also* Chronic health
    problems; Physical health problems
    bereavement and, 179*n*
    care-seeking behavior and, 175*n*
    diary writing and, 74
    immune system and, 19–22
    literature and, 181*n*
    overview, 1–2, 171*n*, 172*n*
    power coping and, 111–112
    psychological links to, 6–10
    secrets and confessions and, 2–6
    social support and, 123
    stress and, 180*n*
    writing to improve outcomes and,
        68–71
Health care utilization, 175*n*
Heart rate. *See also* Cardiovascular
    disease
    expressive writing and, 56–57
    high disclosers versus low disclosers,
        37
    overview, 172*n*
    psychological links to health and
        illness, 9
    stress interview and, 7
HIV/AIDS, 53–54, 63, 174*n*
Hypnotic state, 30–33, 72

Illness prevention, 15–16, 19–22. *See also*
    Health benefits; Physical health
    problems
Immune system, 19–22, 46, 50–54, 94.
    See also Chronic health problems
In-class writing system, 66–68
Inflammation, 50–54, 59. *See also*
    Asthma; Chronic health problems
Inhibition
    benefits of disclosure and, 135
    body's response to confession and,
        34–35
    high disclosers versus low disclosers,
        35–38
    laboratory's role in confession and,
        40–41
    letting-go experience and, 30–33
    physiology of, 33–34
Insight, 28–30
Instant messaging writing, 76
Intellectualism, 77–78
Intensity stage of emotion, 106–109
Intrusive thoughts. *See* Thoughts,
    intrusive and unwanted
Ironic process theory, 84–85, 177*n*.
    See also Thoughts, intrusive and
    unwanted
Irritable bowel syndrome, 52–53

Jealousy, 91
Job loss, 22–23, 140–142
Journaling, ix, 73–75

Language use and development, 70,
    144–146, 150–153, 154
Learning
    in-class writing system and, 66–68
    note-taking and, 71–72, 176*n*
    understanding our world and,
        137–139
    writing and, 68–71, 71–73
Letter writing, 75–76
Letting-go experience, 30–34, 36–37,
    40–41
Lie detection confession effect, 3–5. *See
    also* Confession
Life tasks, 136–137
Life transitions, 69, 110–112, 159–163. *See
    also* Adjustment
Lifestyle, 49–50, 174*n*–175*f*, 175*n*
Linguistic Inquiry and Word Count
    (LIWC) computer program,
    150–152
Listening to disclosures
    burden of, 129–131
    choosing a confidant, 124–129
    nonjudgmental responses and, 125
    overview, 128–129
    values and, 131–132
Logical thinking, 69. *See also* Thinking
    abilities
Loss
    benefit finding and, 143–144
    bereavement and, 104–107
    marital problems following, 120–121
    overview, 178*n*–179*n*
    stress interview and, 7
    when to use or not use expressive
        writing techniques, 160
    writing and, 77
Love, 106–109
Low-level thinking, 87–90, 95, 113. *See
    also* Thinking abilities

Major depressive disorder, 58–60. *See
    also* Depression
Manic depression, 61–62
Marginalized populations, 174*n*
Marital problems, 120–122, 180*n*. *See also*
    Relationship distress
Meaning
    benefit finding and, 143–144
    expressive writing and, 18
    search for, 136–137, 180*n*–181*n*
    understanding our world and,
        137–139

Medication, 80
Memory, 94, 147. *See also* Working
    memory
Mental health, ix–x, 58–62, 173*n*. *See
    also* Bipolar disorder; Chronic
    health problems; Depression;
    Posttraumatic stress disorder
    (PTSD); Psychological factors;
    Schizophrenia
Meta-analytic methods, 24–26
Metabolic risk, 56–57
Mind–body connection, 6
Mindfulness, 90–92, 177*n*–178*n*
Mindlessness, 87–92, 94. *See also*
    Thinking abilities
Music, 148–150, 181*n*

Narrative, 152–153, 157
Negative emotion words, 151. *See also*
    Language use and development
Negative experiences, 161–163
Neuroscience advances, 39
Note taking, 71–72, 176*n*

Obsessions, 93–94. *See also* Thoughts,
    intrusive and unwanted
Occupational factors, 22–23, 140–142
Ongoing crises, 112–113
Online writing, 75–76
Overdisclosing, 78–79

Pain-related disorders, 51–52. *See also*
    Inflammation; Rheumatoid arthritis
Painting, 148–150
Partner-oriented self-regulation, 121
Perseverative cognition, 84. *See also*
    Thoughts, intrusive and unwanted
Personality, 30–33, 74, 165–166
Physical health problems. *See also*
    Chronic health problems; Health
    benefits
  biology and psychology of expressive
      writing and, 46–50
  care-seeking behavior and, 175*n*
  expressive writing and, ix–x, 18
  health behaviors and, 174*n*–175*f*
  illness and health and, 15–16
  immune system and, 19–22
  listening to others' trauma and,
      129–131
  nature of diseases, 44–46
  overview, 172*n*
  psychological links to, 6–10
  secrets and, 2–6, 10–12
  sexual trauma and, 14
  sleep and, 94
  stress and, 180*n*

Physiological reactions
  brain functions and, 38–39
  to confession, 34–35
  discussing trauma and, 29–30
  high disclosers versus low disclosers,
      35–38
  inhibition and confession and, 33–34
  laboratory's role in confession and,
      40–41
  lie detection confession effect and,
      3–5
  overview, 172*n*
Plateau stage of emotion, 106–109
Poetry, 148–150
Polygraph confession effect, 3–5. *See also*
    Confession
Positive emotion words, 151. *See also*
    Language use and development
Positive experiences, 161–163
Posttraumatic stress disorder (PTSD). *See
    also* Mental health; Trauma
  benefit finding and, 143–144
  discussing the trauma, 29–30
  expressive writing and, ix–x, 60–61,
      63, 173*n*
  HIV/AIDS and, 54
  resilience and, 100–101
  thought cycles and, 85, 177*n*
  translating experiences into language,
      144–146
Power, 128
Power coping, 96–97, 106–109, 110–114
Prevention, illness. *See* Illness prevention
Problem-solving skills
  benefit finding and, 144
  leaning and health outcomes and, 69
  mindfulness and, 90
  writing and, 72–73
Process writing, 70–71. *See also*
    Freewriting
Professional help
  bereavement and, 104
  choosing a confidant and, 126–127
  coping with trauma and, 101–103
  disclosure and, 181*n*–182*n*
  listening to others' trauma and,
      130–131
  overview, 169–170
  transference and, 127
Pronoun use in writing, 151–152. *See also*
    Language use and development
Psychological factors, 6–12, 171*n*. *See also*
    Mental health
Psychosomatics, 5–11, 44–46
Psychotherapy
  bereavement and, 104
  choosing a confidant and, 126–127

disclosure and, 181n–182n
expressive writing and, 173n–174n
listening to others' trauma and,
    130–131
transference and, 127
trauma and, 101–103

Reading skills, 69–71
Relationship distress, 121–122, 159–161,
    179n, 180n. See also Marital
    problems
Relaxation therapy, 19
Religion, 138, 164
Resilience, 100–101
Resolution, 136–137
Respiratory changes, 5, 6, 7, 8–9, 43, 45
Rheumatoid arthritis, 43, 51–52, 63.
    See also Autoimmune disorders;
    Chronic health problems;
    Inflammation
Rumination, 83–85, 93–94, 136–137,
    176n–177n. See also Thoughts,
    intrusive and unwanted

Scheduling of expressive writing
    sessions, 163–164, 166–167. See also
    Expressive writing technique
Schizophrenia, 61–62
Secrets. See also Disclosure
    benefits of disclosure and, 27–30, 135
    choosing a confidant, 128–129
    diary writing and, 74–75
    disease and, 48
    health and, 2–6
    overview, 1–2, 10–12
    social support and, 116–117, 180n
Self-absorption, 79
Self-care, 49–50
Self-compassion, 91–92
Self-esteem, 122–123
Self-expression, 148, 148–150, 181n
Self-help literature, 12
Self-kindness, 91
Self-knowledge, 5–6
Self-reflection
    altering thinking styles to avoid,
        89–90
    coping with trauma and, 114
    disclosure and, 140–142
    unwanted thoughts and, 94–95
    values and, 133–134
    writing and, 77–79
Sexual trauma, 13–15, 139–140
Shame, 40, 91
Sleep, 93–94, 153–154, 160, 178n
Social connections, 153–154
Social factors, 47–48

Social media writing, 75–76, 176n
Social support. See also Friendship
    choosing a confidant, 124–129
    disclosure process model and, 157
    listening to others' trauma, 129–131
    loss of following a death, 118–120
    overview, 115–117, 180n
    talking about and reacting to trauma
        and, 117–118
    values and, 131–132
    when its helpful versus not helpful,
        122–123
    working memory and, 154
Spacing of expressive writing sessions,
    163–164, 166–167. See also
    Expressive writing technique
Speaking voice, 30–31
Stages of coping, 98–99. See also Coping
Standard expressive writing, 163. See also
    Expressive writing technique
Stigmatized populations, 174n
Story writing, 148–150, 152–153
Stress
    altering thinking styles to avoid,
        87–90
    depression and, 59
    diary writing and, 74–75
    disease and, 46–47, 180n
    listening to others' trauma and,
        129–131
    nature of diseases and, 45–46
    secrets and, 10–11
    self-care and, 49–50
    summarizing and sharing memory to
        reduce, 147
    suppression of thoughts and, 84
    unwanted thoughts and, 94–95
Stress hormones, 46–47
Stress interview, 6–7, 29–30
Substance use, 89–90
Suicide, 97–98, 119–120
Summary, 147, 176n
Support following trauma, 101–103,
    115–117. See also Coping; Social
    support
Support groups, 119–120
suppression of thoughts, 81–85. See also
    Thoughts, intrusive and unwanted

Technology, 75–76, 150–152, 176n
Therapy
    benefit finding and, 144
    bereavement and, 104
    choosing a confidant and, 126–127
    coping with trauma and, 101–103
    disclosure and, 181n–182n
    expressive writing and, 173n–174n

Therapy (*cont.*)
  listening to disclosures and, 125,
    130–131
  overview, 169–170
  transference and, 127
  writing as a replacement for, 80
Thinking abilities. *See also* Thoughts,
    intrusive and unwanted
  altering thinking styles to avoid stress
    and, 87–90
  healthy versus unhealthy ways to
    think and, 85–87
  leaning and health outcomes and, 69
  mindfulness and, 90–92
  secrets and, 10–11
  summarizing and sharing memory
    and, 147
  training of, 69–71
Thinking words, 151. *See also* Language
    use and development
Thoughts, intrusive and unwanted.
    See also Obsessions; Rumination;
    Thinking abilities
  altering thinking styles to avoid stress
    and, 87–90
  anxiety and depression and, 92
  healthier thinking, 85–87
  life tasks and, 136–137
  mindfulness and, 90–92
  overview, 81–85, 94–95, 177n
  sleep and, 93–94
Timing of expressive writing sessions,
    163–164, 168. *See also* Expressive
    writing technique
Topic cueing, 32–33
Topic of writing, 167–168. *See also*
    Expressive writing technique
Topics, sequence of, 32–33
Transference, 127
Transitions, life, 69, 110–112, 159–163.
    See also Adjustment
Trauma. *See also* Coping; Posttraumatic
    stress disorder (PTSD)
  benefit finding and, 143–144
  bereavement and, 104–107
  brain functions and, 38–39
  coping with, 179n
  diary writing and, 74–75
  disclosure process model and, 154–157
  discussing, 27–28, 29–30
  expressive writing and, 17–19, 77,
    159–161, 167–168
  finding meaning in, 138–139
  focusing on in expressive writing,
    161–163
  immune system and, 20–22
  leaning and health outcomes and, 69
  life tasks and, 136–137

listening to others' trauma, 129–131
listening to others' trauma and,
    117–118
marital problems following, 120–121
psychotherapy and, 101–103
resilience and, 100–101
role of narrative and, 152–153
stress interview and, 7
talking about and reacting to, 117–118
talking about and reacting to trauma
    and, 129–131
translating experiences into language,
    144–146
traumatic sexual experiences, 13–15
understanding and, 139–140,
    180n–181n
Traumatic grief, 105, 110, 113–114. *See
    also* Bereavement; Grief; Loss;
    Trauma
Trust, 124–126, 128–129, 131–132
Type 2 diabetes. *See* Diabetes

Understanding
  benefit finding and, 143–144
  disclosure and, 140–142
  example of, 140–142
  need for, 137
  overview, 137–139, 180n–181n
  translating experiences into language,
    144–146
  the unfathomable, 139–140
Unwanted thoughts. *See* Thoughts,
    intrusive and unwanted

Values, 18, 131–134, 143–144
Voice, 30–33
Vulnerability, 40, 124

Where to write, 168. *See also* Expressive
    writing technique
"White bear dilemma," 84. *See also*
    Thoughts, intrusive and unwanted
Wishful thinking, 95
Word use, 150–152. *See also* Language use
    and development
Working memory. *See also* Memory
  altering thinking styles to avoid stress
    and, 88–90
  disclosure process model and, 156, 157
  leaning and health outcomes and,
    68–69
  mindfulness and, 90–91
  overview, 153–154
  testing, 86–87
  translating experiences into language
    and, 153–154
  when to use or not use expressive
    writing techniques, 160

Working through stage of coping, 99. *See also* Coping
Wound healing, 46–47, 172*n*
Writing. *See also* Expressive writing technique
  diary writing and, 73–75
  downside of, 76–79
  education benefits of, 66–71
  leaning and health outcomes and, 68–71
  overview, 79–80
  self-expression and, 148
  social media writing, 75–76
  summarizing and sharing memory and, 147
  translating experiences into language, 150–152
Writing skills, 69–71
Writing style, 31–33

About the Authors

James W. Pennebaker, PhD, the originator of expressive writing, is Regents Centennial Professor of Psychology at the University of Texas at Austin. Dr. Pennebaker conducts award-winning research and has published numerous books on the links between expressive writing and physical and mental health.

Joshua M. Smyth, PhD, is Professor of Biobehavioral Health and of Medicine at The Pennsylvania State University. Dr. Smyth has conducted extensive research on expressive writing and other innovative methods for promoting health and well-being and coping with stress.